EMMA JANE UNSWORTH is
and screenwriter. Her first nove
motion picture, for which Unsv
The film premiered at Sundance Film Festival 20..,.
writes for television and various magazines. Her latest novel,
Adults, has been heralded as 'hilarious' (Dolly Alderton),
'tender' (Jessie Burton) and 'dazzling' (Marian Keyes) and
was a *Sunday Times* bestseller.

PRAISE FOR *AFTER THE STORM*

'A compulsive read, one that any mother will
recognise parts of herself within, even if she has
not, like Unsworth, experienced brutal PND'
IRISH INDEPENDENT

'A call to arms to centre the mental health of new
mothers and push back against the taboos that force
so many to feel they must suffer in silence'
REFINERY29

'Postnatal depression is not supposed to make you
laugh, but brutal honesty and dazzling humour are
part of Emma Jane Unsworth's award-winning literary
arsenal … Her first foray into non-fiction is a brave
and compelling part-memoir, part-manifesto'
MARIE CLAIRE

'Oh, what a book'
STYLIST

After the Storm

Postnatal Depression and the
Utter Weirdness of New Motherhood

EMMA JANE
UNSWORTH

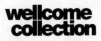

PROFILE BOOKS

This paperback edition first published in 2022

First published in Great Britain in 2021 by
PROFILE BOOKS LTD
29 Cloth Fair
London ECIA 7JQ
www.profilebooks.com

Published in association with Wellcome Collection

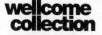

183 Euston Road
London NWI 2BE
www.wellcomecollection.org

Part of the Wellcome Collection Life Lines series: today's finest
storytellers on health and being human.

1 3 5 7 9 10 8 6 4 2

Typeset in Garamond by MacGuru Ltd
Printed and bound in Great Britain by CPI Group (UK) Ltd, Croydon, CRO 4YY

The moral right of the author has been asserted.

A CIP catalogue record for this book is available from the British Library.

ISBN 978 1 78816 655 3
eISBN 978 1 78283 769 5

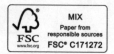

Contents

In snowfall, I haunted Motherhood's cemeteries,
the sweet fallen beneath my feet –
Our Lady of the Birth Trauma, Our Lady of Psychosis.
I wanted to speak to them, tell them I understood,
but the words came out scrambled, so I knelt instead
and prayed in the chapel of Motherhood, prayed
for that whole wild fucking queendom,
its sorrow, its unbearable skinless beauty,
and all the souls that were in it. I prayed and prayed
until my voice was a nightcry,
sunlight pixellating my face like a kaleidoscope.

from 'The Republic of Motherhood', Liz Berry

For Ian and LF
– and for wild queens, everywhere

The Cloud

It is the worst of times and the worst of times. Brighton, May 2017. I am bone-tired, shoving a buggy through jostling crowds. Early summer sun beats down from a blue sky. People are eating ice creams and sitting in deck chairs, enjoying the year's first blast of warmth. But this is no ordinary Sunday on the seafront. Either side of me, two lines of polished parked cars – all Minis – stretch for ever into the distance. There are Minis in every possible colour and style. Some are themed like cartoon characters or sporting heroes. Some have eyelashes. Some have stickers on the bonnet and furry seats inside. Hundreds of people walk – no, amble – in between, admiring the cars. The flow of the crowd is one-way. I am trapped. On I trudge, trying not to run over any feet/children/dogs, trying not to make eye contact with the smiling faces, the shiny, happy people basking in the Mini Love.

I had set out from my flat not knowing where I was going, just needing to walk, to get out, to put one foot in front of the other, to do something that felt vaguely autonomous. These walks are the only choice I have left. I slammed the door, cursed the never-arriving lift (No. 1 Bane of My Life), crossed the road, crossed the perilous cycle path, cursed at a cyclist (Bane No. 2), and turned left along the front. I stomped along the promenade – past the i360 viewing

1

tower, past the seafood shacks and the smokehouse, the ice-cream stalls, past the pier, lit up and heaving, past the crazy golf and the aquarium. Brighton is a place where people come for holidays, for hen-dos and high-jinks. It's a place of merriment and celebration. I am a dark cloud over it. My partner, Ian, actually said that to me this morning. 'It's like living with a dark cloud.' He has said kind things, too. He mostly says kind things. He is a man at the end of his rope.

I know that I have not been easy to live with for a while now. My mind has been steadily darkening since December, a month or so after the baby was born. I have accumulated layer upon layer of bad feeling; of negativity, rage and doom. I am swollen with it, waiting to explode. 'I think you have postnatal depression,' Ian says regularly. 'I think you should go and talk to someone. A therapist. Your GP.'

He is a GP two days a week. He is a graphic novelist and writer the rest of the time. Even though I got him to check all of my moles the first time we were in bed together (apparently this happens to doctors a *lot*), I am refusing to accept his diagnosis on this one. I don't feel depressed. I feel fucking furious. To make matters worse, in my hazy state of mind I have inadvertently stumbled into the midst of the London to Brighton Mini Run, an annual get-together for Mini owners. The smell of petrol hangs in the air. People have dolled up for the occasion. They smoke rollies and cheers tinnies. There is a distinct festival vibe. A cruel pastiche of my former life. I used to go to festivals. I was last woman standing at many of them, greeting the dawn with a can of lager and a wide grin. Now I can hardly stand up straight.

I am running on adrenaline. Or rather, the fumes of adrenaline. I haven't had more than four hours of sleep in a row for seven months. I am jumpy and twitchy, like a person on high alert. I want to shout and scream and lie down and curl into a ball and have someone – anyone – just take the baby for a few hours and give me time to regroup my thoughts. I feel like I am on the edge of a psychotic fit; some uncontrollable outburst. Ian has told me he is worried I am 'almost psychotic' more than once. But I have no options. I feel like I should just be getting on with this. Surely not everyone can find it this hard, or humans … just wouldn't do it, would they? So here I am, almost psychotic, surrounded by jolly Mods and Minis – my least favourite car.

Ian and I have a Mini. It is an old pigeon-coloured thing with one functioning door. The electrics are bust so the windows don't open. Pieces of the upholstery and dashboard keep falling off. Ian and I argue every time we try and get into (or out of) it. The passenger door has been broken for two years but it will cost more to get it fixed than the car is worth. Getting a baby in and out is a gymnastic feat. I often end up literally on my arse in the street, baby held aloft, bags scattered. Travelling 300 miles to see Ian's or my relatives, in Manchester and Wales respectively, is a logistical nightmare. Ian refuses to get rid of the Mini (he's had it ten years), and I see this as him digging his heels in as some kind of eternal bachelor, in denial about his new responsibilities. The Mini convention is like something sent from my subconscious to mock me. And I can't get out. It's like a bad dream. (I remember those, from the days when I used to sleep.) People must be wondering why I'm charging ahead with such a thunderous look on my face. My phone vibrates in my pocket. I have it on silent so as not to wake the baby in the precious moments that he sleeps. I miss calls, but then people are calling less.

My whole life has become one of shutting down, switching off, of retreating into darkness.

It's a text, from Ian. 'Where are you?'

I text him back. It's hard to type while walking and steering. He's worried, but I also want to vent at him. I am the master of angry texts, especially angry nocturnal texts when he is away. (How come he gets to go away?)

I am stuck in the middle of a Mini convention

I wait a moment, and then I launch my irresistible punchline:

And I fucking hate Minis

He doesn't rise to it, not today. I half expect him to. He'd love it here. He'd blend right in. Not like me, with my three-day-old clothes and scraped-up hair and foul demeanour. He texts back. I look, expecting some lengthy and passionate defence of his beloved Minis, but no. He says:

I'm going to get on my bike and meet you at the marina

I do not reply. I do not look for him up on the cycle path (although he will have to pass me up there, where the traffic is moving freely, unlike the slow, aching meander of the Mini convention). I stomp on. Everyone and everything is in my way. Sunday is in my way. Life is in my way. By the time I get to the marina I am a ball of rage, some kind of dying earthbound sun, a red giant on her way out. We buy burgers. As we sit down, where it is quieter, the baby wakes and looks at me. My heart pounds in my chest, as it does in the night, as it does any time he might need me. I pull out his bottle. The baby accepts the bottle and sucks on it. The knot in my chest – the constant knot of anxiety – slackens off a little. The baby is okay. Don't panic.

I begin to eat. I chomp on the burger joylessly, not tasting it, hawking and squeezing it down my dry throat. My love for food – like my love for most things – has mostly disappeared. I eat whole packs of biscuits, mindlessly, to stay awake in the afternoon. I shovel in jumbo bars of chocolate, barely chewing. Sugar is my fix – but also, I sense a self-destruction in these acts, beyond any previous joyous self-destruction: a self-loathing I have never known the like of before. A darkness that is opening and widening, dividing the centre of me.

Ian watches me eat. I shake my head and scowl. I don't want to be watched. Don't want to be scrutinised. Leave me alone in my … My brain says it before I consciously allow it to: *Misery.* And there it is.

Boom.

I am miserable.

And I know it.

I start to cry. Ian nods and hugs me.

'I think I might be depressed,' I say.

'Yes. Will you go and see someone?'

'I'll go and see someone for a potential diagnosis,' I say.

His face sort of crumples, but it's all I can give him right now. I am so ashamed. The floodgates have opened and I can't stop crying. How did this happen? I am tough. I am smart. I have built a career. I have lived alone. I have spent decades carving out a life for myself that feels right and fulfilling. Now I am cracking, right down the middle.

A Uniquely
Vulnerable Time

A lot has changed since then. For a start, I don't hate Minis any more. I actually thank them, in part, for pushing me to some kind of breaking point. Crying in a burger restaurant is never a good look, but it was a good thing I cracked, really. I needed to so that I could admit what was happening and start rebuilding my life. Even though I was so afraid – so afraid – of saying I needed help, because somehow I knew that by saying it, the whole thing would come crumbling down.

Many things were walling me in, separating me from the truth. Pride, shame, a deep fear of failure. I felt like I was the only person doing it wrong. The only person feeling it wrong. I felt as though anything less than perfect was wrong. In fact, what I went through wasn't so unusual.

According to the NHS, more than 1 in 10 women experience postnatal depression (PND), and it is thought many more cases go unreported. Women are too often afraid or ashamed to speak up or admit there is a problem. I was hesitant to write this book because I thought, *What if my son reads it in ten years and gets upset, or thinks I didn't love him in the beginning?* But as my devastatingly wise friend Katie says:

'People don't have babies; they have people.' My son will have his own opinions one day, and I hope we can have conversations about it and he'll understand that I'm doing this for all the women who might be struggling and don't know how to say. All the women who don't know what the hell is wrong with them, like I didn't.

What is PND, exactly? Well, that's a huge question (welcome to my book!) and, like most mental health issues, is slightly different for everyone. According to the World Health Organisation, postnatal depression ('postpartum depression' in the United States) is:

> A syndrome associated with pregnancy or the puerperium (commencing within about 6 weeks after delivery) that involves significant mental and behavioural features, most commonly depressive symptoms. The syndrome does not include delusions, hallucinations, or other psychotic symptoms. This designation should not be used to describe mild and transient depressive symptoms that do not meet the diagnostic requirements for a depressive episode, which may occur soon after delivery (so-called postpartum blues).

It's likely something women have always experienced, although historically little has been written about it. Hippocrates described the emotional difficulties of the postpartum period, writing about 'puerperal fever' which produced delirium, agitation and bouts of mania. However, a mother's mental health before and after giving birth has generally not been of great concern, or has been classified out of existence by being lumped in with other mental illnesses.

In the nineteenth century, Charlotte Perkins Gilman's semi-autobiographical story 'The Yellow Wallpaper' featured a woman diagnosed with nervous depression after the birth of her first child. Confined to one room as a 'rest cure', she becomes fixated on the wallpaper and convinced that a woman is trapped behind it. The story ends with her attempting to release the woman by tearing the wallpaper down – clawing at her cage, effectively.

Professor Hilary Marland has extensively researched the treatment and perception of women's mental health in the nineteenth and early twentieth centuries. In Victorian times, postnatal mental illness was often written off as just 'insanity'. Professor Marland describes some haunting examples, including the case of Mary Sibbald, who was admitted to the Royal Edinburgh Asylum in 1855 'suffering from puerperal insanity',

> one of a number of patients who were reported as being too demented to describe their condition. Noted to be incoherent, violent and thin on admission, Mary had no milk and was unable to feed her child. She was very disruptive and turned her room 'upside down', but at the same time was described as exhausted, pale and weak, with a feeble pulse, dull-eyed and showing 'symptoms of sinking from condition'. An abscess on her left breast was poulticed, she was given brandy and morphine and force-fed custard and sherry.

Force-fed custard and sherry. Maybe I should have tried that.

Early motherhood is always hard, and I'm sure many of the symptoms I describe in this book will echo the experiences of all new mums. Childbirth and the first six months are often so traumatic I think women should be screened like soldiers who have come back from war. Public discourse about postnatal trauma is steadily growing, and hurray for that, but we still don't talk about motherhood honestly enough in the mainstream. Nothing prepares you for the onslaught, exhaustion and anxiety.

So how do you know if you've actually got PND? There is no physical test, but there are questionnaires used by doctors to work towards a diagnosis. A GP in the UK might use the PHQ-9 and GAD-7 questionnaires, which provide depression and anxiety scores. But half the women who suffer a peri- or postnatal illness don't disclose. I didn't. This is sometimes due to fear, but not always. Sometimes you're just clueless and lost through no fault of your own. If all your usual reference points and life norms have gone, and everyone's experience – and baby – is different, how can you even tell when you need help? It's difficult to know what to look for, and differentiate between the 'normal' weird as opposed to a problematic weird. Because *everything* is suddenly weird.

Dr Rebecca Moore, a British perinatal psychiatrist with over twenty years' experience of working with women during pregnancy and the postpartum period, gives some insight as to why women might not reach out when they're struggling. 'It can be hard to tease out, especially if it's your first baby,' she explains.

> It's hard to know whether you're just feeling knackered. We all have bad days where everything seems to go wrong and we feel really low. The thing to bear in mind is how often things are happening. If you're having an

occasional low day that's probably just the way it goes for many women. But if every day is feeling bad for most of the day, then I think that's something different. If [every day] you're feeling really anxious or low or can't sleep and you don't want to see anybody, then, if you feel able to talk to somebody about it, you should. It's about how much it's impacting on you.

But doesn't this request for self-diagnosis make it yet another job for women to do when they're already maxed out? It requires a leap of faith to make any kind of call. 'Sometimes we can't see it ourselves, but our partners can, or parents can, or friends can,' Dr Moore says.

Part of the problem is we're always asking women to 'reach out' and often they don't feel able to and don't know where to go, or might feel judged. As a society we need to be better at reaching out and checking in on our friends, rather than them having to source their own care at a time when they feel really awful. In my opinion, the way services are set up is the wrong way around. We wait for people to be at breaking point, but we don't capture the track up to it. A lot of that has come through stresses and strains in health visiting – they are not able to provide that 'listening' support they once would have done where they would have picked up on more cases. There has been a decimation of children's centres, which for a lot of people would have been a lifeline of support. So you've got this erosion of these kinds of things that did provide that help for people with a milder presentation.

Coronavirus has only made things worse. Dr Moore says the figures for PND 'skyrocketed' in 2020. During the pandemic, women's choices in birth altered very quickly: home-birth teams shut down; partners weren't allowed to appointments. There's no doubt that a bad experience of childbirth can drastically affect mental health. Dr Moore is co-founder of a national collective of experts on birth trauma: Make Birth Better. A lot of the women she's worked with over the years were mentally well but the thing that tipped them over was their birth experience. 'Childbirth is a uniquely vulnerable time for women and is tied up with women's rights and the notion of consent.' It definitely triggered mental illness in me. I'd never had depression before, and I wasn't depressed during my pregnancy, but childbirth was where everything started to go wrong.

I want to rewind a bit before that, though, and talk about pregnancy – because that was when my autonomy and confidence first started to take a battering. It blew my mind that my body was growing another body. (Inside! Like a meaty Russian doll!) But I also started to become aware that I had a mystery inside me; a mystery that other people – often complete strangers – felt able to take ownership of.

Comedy Sketch Idea

A pregnant woman in a café orders a coffee. Another woman next to her pipes up: 'I hope that's decaf!'

'Why?'

Other Woman nods to Pregnant Woman's stomach. Pregnant Woman shakes her head.

'Oh, I'm not pregnant.'

Other Woman looks surprised.

'It's a tumour. Inoperable. I have three weeks to live.'

Other Woman's face falls. 'Oh god, I'm so sorry.'

'Yeah. It's breaking my family's heart. Coffee's about the only thing getting me through.'

Other Woman takes her coffee and leaves. Pregnant Woman smiles an evil smile. Milks her coffee.

The Mountain

When I was pregnant I was obsessed with watching YouTube videos of people summitting the world's highest mountains. I had a particular, slightly twisted penchant for the disaster movie *Everest*. I fantasised a lot about the Highlands of Scotland, a place I have always gone for solace, thinking time and to feel like myself – usually in a motorhome for weeks on end. I was afraid to go now. I found myself fearful of the smallest expeditions. Train journeys, flights, fast-food outlets. My natural intrepidness was diminished. So, I watched other people climb mountains on TV instead. At the time I didn't make the connection between the growing peak around my middle and the huge feat before me. Besides, I hardly felt like Atlas.

You hear about women being touched, unasked. No one petted my bump inappropriately, but I often felt infantilised. And the sad subtext of that kind of treatment is that you are simply not to be trusted with the job in the hand. There was the waiter in the hotel who refused to serve me cooked mussels, even though I got the NHS website up on my phone and showed him it was perfectly safe for pregnant women to eat cooked shellfish, just not raw. 'No,' he said, 'Chef won't do it. Chef's wife is a midwife.' Wow. I was being double-mansplained. Whether this was true or not, I didn't feel I could investigate, so instead I grumpily ordered some depressing penne and a glass of white wine – which I expected him to refuse too, but no! He gave me wine. Evil wine. They can be terribly inconsistent, the pregnancy police.

There was the midwife who made me blow into a carbon-monoxide test even though she'd asked me whether I'd stopped smoking and I'd told her I had. This was true – I hadn't had a single puff since I'd found out I was pregnant. I just hadn't fancied it. But lo and behold, the carbon-monoxide test beeped away like I was a regular Fag Ash Lil. 'Let me do it again,' I said, the swot in me rising. I hated failing tests. I did it again. The alarm said I contained too much carbon monoxide. 'You try it,' I said to Ian, who'd come with me to the appointment and has never smoked a cigarette in his life. He blew into the tube. Nada. Clean as a whistle. So it couldn't even be that we had carbon monoxide in the flat. 'I must just be a toxic person,' I said. 'Hmm,' said the midwife. I could tell she thought I was still smoking. I obsessed over it at home, and the next time I went to see her, when she asked me to blow into the test again, I refused. I said I didn't want to contribute to the local trust's data at the expense of my wellbeing. She was fine about it.

It's funny, how it begins – the combination of being made to feel like you should be able to do everything – it's all so easy! Modern women can have it all! – and yet simultaneously be made to feel incapable, scared, doubting of yourself. As someone who was thirty-seven and relatively good at managing my own life and judging situations, I started to feel shaken. I couldn't see it at the time, but now when I look back I see how there was a front-facing part of pregnancy

– the shopfront, if you will – where it was important to seem in control and appreciative of feminism's benefits; I took pride in this. And then there was a back room, a storeroom of feelings, where worries and inadequacies swirled.

As well as infantilised, I often felt disrespected.

There was the Hooray Henry on the train from London to Brighton who refused to give me his seat when I asked for it because I was feeling sick. I was wearing a Baby on Board badge, which seemed to irk him. 'Where is your baby?' he said. 'Did you lose it?' The people around him squirmed. I felt like saying, *Are you referring to my previous miscarriage?* But I don't think he'd have got the joke. I stared at him, incredulous that someone could – in public, in daylight, in 2016 – be such a total cunt. He wasn't deterred. He sat his ground. A woman by the window, the kindest woman in the world, in the shortest denim hotpants, got up and offered me a fig from a paper bag. 'Have my seat,' she said. I thanked her and sat down. When we reached her stop she smiled at me, touched my shoulder and walked away, and I watched the brown slashes of her buttocks moving under ripped denim. I was madly in love with her. Still am. I hope I see her again one day. I would like to give her a bag of figs. I would like to tell her that she reminded me that kindness is the default setting for humans. I would like to tell her that, in my hardest, meanest moments, the thought of her has stopped me going postal.

There was the man who tried to run me over for a parking space when I was eight months pregnant. I was waiting by the side of the road outside the hospital while Ian turned the cursed Mini around and came back. A man pulled up wanting the space. I explained my husband was about to

come and park in it. He said, 'Well he's not here now, is he?'
I moved forward into the space. The man began to move
his car towards me, into the space. I had to move out of the
way before he ran me over. The woman in the passenger seat
of his car had her head in her hands. I wonder what sort of
private agonies she was going through at home, living with a
man like that. As he got out of the car, I took out my phone
and started photographing him and the number plate. God
knows what I was planning to do with the photos, but it's
the modern way, isn't it. 'OH YOU'RE PHOTOGRAPH-
ING ME, YOU'RE PHOTOGRAPHING ME!' he shouted.
'TAKE SOME MORE.'

I present this catalogue of fuckery firstly to show the kind
of shit that pregnant women have to deal with, and secondly
to remind myself of the chipping away that had begun of my
self-worth and judgement.

And then of course there's coffee. For a bullshit-stripping
read that really cuts through the contradictory information
pregnant women are bombarded with, I recommend *Expecting Better* by Emily Oster. Oster is an economist who, when
she was expecting her first child, found herself confused by
conflicting information about what pregnant women should
and shouldn't do, and as a result powerless to make the right
decisions. So she applied her economist's tools to the available statistics and compiled a book that debunks the myths
and sheds light on the safety of things like alcohol, caffeine,
home birth and various other 'mysteries'. Her conclusion
on alcohol: 'There is no good evidence that light drinking
during pregnancy negatively impacts your baby. You should
be comfortable with: up to one drink a day in the second
and third trimesters; one to two drinks a week in the first

trimester.' On caffeine: 'In moderation, caffeine is fine. All evidence supports having up to two cups [a day].' And on smoking: 'Smoking during pregnancy is dangerous for your baby.' Check it out. I found the book really enlightening and empowering. Shame I only discovered it during my second long-term pregnancy and not my first.

And while we're on the subject of things I wish I'd known first time round …

In May 2020, ten weeks into my fifth pregnancy (I want to acknowledge the three that didn't work out, in addition to the first one that stuck around and resulted in my son's birth), a kind and brilliant midwife called Didi told me at my booking appointment, eyes smiling above her corona mask, that I should be careful about reducing my anti-depressants during pregnancy because at twenty-six weeks women experience a surge of cortisol, which helps get the baby's lungs ready for the outside world, including the possibility of a premature birth. The effect of that cortisol surge on the woman is heightened anxiety.

I had never, ever heard about this before. But it feels pretty significant. I remember during the pregnancy with my son feeling very stressed around that time, and taking it out on Ian and, often, wayward cyclists on the cycle path outside my house who refused to stop at the pedestrian crossing. I may have yelled at a few. How many other things like this, how many hormone surges and brain spurts, might it help women to know about and prepare for? When people talk about the 'baby blues' it's vague, and sounds trivial – pretty, almost. A colour you might paint the nursery. But there are huge changes occurring within women's brains during pregnancy and early motherhood – changes we know astonishingly little about. The pregnancy 'week-by-week' diagrams show women's bodies from the neck down. We are literally decapitated into unthinking vessels. In fact, women's brains change more drastically and quickly during pregnancy and early motherhood than during any other period of their lives – including puberty.

Scientists can't yet say how maternal brain changes interact with things like sleep deprivation or trauma, which many women experience during childbirth. Or poverty, or abuse, which many women experience alongside motherhood. Importantly, they can't yet say whether postpartum mood disorders are the result of something gone awry in typical changes to a mother's brain, or whether they are caused by a triggering of other brain circuitry.

One in five women will have some form of mental illness during pregnancy or the postpartum period, according to a 2017 study by the Royal College of Obstetricians and Gynaecologists. But even when it doesn't tip over into illness, the brain changes are vast. In an article for the Boston Globe in 2018, Chelsea Conaboy reports that the flood of hormones women experience during pregnancy, childbirth and breastfeeding (should they choose to do it) 'primes the brain for dramatic change in regions thought to make up the "maternal circuit". Affected brain regions include those that enable a mother to multitask to meet baby's needs, help her to empathise with her infant's pain and emotions, and regulate how she responds to positive stimuli (such as baby's coo) or to perceived threats.'

Could this help to explain the heightened anxiety many new mothers feel? The forgetfulness of some things and the hypervigilance when it comes to others? The unmooring from our sense of identity?

Dr Jodi Pawluski is a Canadian neuroscientist and thera-pist who has extensively studied what she calls the 'neglected neuroscience' of the maternal brain, working largely with mice. (Turns out there are ethics when it comes to exper-imenting on human mothers, who knew?) I ask her what she thinks about the decapitated diagrams. 'YES!' she says. 'Where are all the heads?' She goes on to tell me that there is an overall decrease in grey-matter volume during pregnancy and the postpartum period – but that's not necessarily a bad thing. She urges me to think of it as more of a 'fine tuning' instead. And while there is a decrease in neurogenesis (the making of new brain cells), which has been associated with forgetfulness, it's maybe not so much about lack of new neurons than the existing neurons functioning more effi-ciently. Simply put: parts of the brain become more precise in function. These parts have been called 'the maternal circuit'. 'With modern imaging we have seen certain parts of women's brains activated when babies cry, or when they see pictures of babies,' she says. 'The maternal circuit is different brain areas that are usually parts of other circuits but that come together and work together to mediate parental behaviours and proper parental responses.'

The work of Elseline Hoekzema at Leiden university in 2017 and 2019 shows that the decrease in volume of these brain regions is not associated with memory changes (at least not the memory types they looked at) but, in fact, with feelings of maternal attachment. So a lower volume of these brain areas correlate with greater feelings of attachment. As Dr Pawluski puts it: 'Less is more when it comes to the brain and maternal care-giving.'

It is thought that the grey matter returns after a couple

of years. I felt this was true to my experience, and found the science so reassuring. Wouldn't it be great if there was a week-by-week diagram of pregnant women's brain changes alongside the diagrams of their bodies and the baby's development, so that we might know what to expect? So we could see which weeks we might feel a certain way, as well as discovering all the details about how big our bump will be, or which week the baby gets eyelashes, or starts drinking its own pee? If I'd known there were massive brain changes afoot – if I'd known that unfamiliar emotions are part of a *healthy* experience of new motherhood – it might not have felt as much like my fault, or my failing when they tipped over into something else. If we cut through the golden mythology and romanticism and show how the changes women experience are biological, not constitutional, then we might find that postnatal mental illness has, one day, more targeted diagnosis and treatment. Even considering a range of feelings for a typical pre- and postpartum experience is radical right now. It's not all lovely-lovely-huggy-huggy – a lot of it is just weird, new and hard. Maybe if I'd known this, I wouldn't have been so blindsided by it all.

'There's a normal range of brain changes and feelings – and it's not all happy,' says Dr Pawluski. 'When it persists and you can't function then this is not healthy. But there is a normal range of emotions that need to be talked about and that are healthy to have.'

I tell a friend excitedly about these findings. 'But would you have wanted to know?' she asks. To which I answer a resounding '*Yes!*' Everyone is different, but I want to be realistically informed. The idea that women can't handle the truth of their experiences is a dangerous and pervasive one.

There is a huge reluctance to allow any negative thinking about motherhood. I was irked by the PR-sheeny bullshit that painted, from the start, a perfect depiction of motherhood and nicey-niceness that made me personally feel utterly unprepared for childbirth and the aftermath. I'm all for positive thinking. But, you know, laced with a good dose of reality. It's not gloomy to recognise that a huge thing can comprise bad as well as good, is it? But where babies are involved it's like we've got to slap on a rictus grin and chant, Everything's lovely! Which is dangerous on so many levels. I made a cocaine joke at pregnancy yoga (*that* went down like a lead balloon, let me tell you). I won't even tell you about going on a weaning course when I was hungover. All I will say is: purée and poo are not what you want to ponder at those times. Just call me the queen of baby-group faux pas.

Why are there so many taboos? Why does pregnancy have to be perfect or bust? The mandatory twelve weeks of silence at the start of a pregnancy seems so damaging, for example. I know that this period of silence isolated me in the false shame of my first miscarriage. Silencing women through their reproductive experience seems to prevent so much useful information about the realities of fertility getting out.

For society, for the patriarchy, and crucially the capitalism that is symbiotic with it, it is useful to preserve the façade that motherhood is blissful. It keeps women doing it. It keeps them buying stuff to do it 'right'. It keeps them buying things to quell the anxiety. And, ultimately, it keeps them feeling inadequate and inferior. During that pregnancy I was certainly busy beavering away at my little shopfront. I bought all the right things: the best cot, the fashionable buggy, even a weird vaginal exercise balloon to stop me tearing, the 'Epi-no'

– as in: 'Say NO to that episiotomy!' (For the blissfully igno-
rant, an episiotomy is when they cut you open at your vagina
so that you don't split along your entire perineum.)

But in the back, in the storeroom of my anxieties, my
true feelings were brewing. And I might as well have stuck
that blue balloon somewhere else for all the good it did.

Red Shift

My baby blazed out of me in less than three hours. This was not a desirably 'fast' birth. This was an evacuation. My body wanted this baby *out*. The doctors and midwives were overwhelmed. I was stratospheric with pain. Years later I remember that day – that day I went to war with my body, against my body, for my body – as the closest I've come to death. That experience took its toll. It was a challenge, and one I wasn't up to; one that arguably I could not possibly be up to, being so ill-prepared mentally and practically – because I had been made to feel it would be a breeze. I was like someone who had been sent up Everest with a pair of tennis shoes and a 'Keep Calm and Drink Decaf' t-shirt. I recall the jolly NCT classes, where I wore my light cynicism like armour, without knowing how much I really needed to protect myself.

Tuesday 8 November 2016. A day of very bad and very good things. Donald Trump took the White House, Leonard Cohen died, and my son was born. (We were hoping he'd be the reincarnation, but then I read that LC had vowed to come back as his daughter's dog. Better luck next time.) The maternity ward was on the eleventh floor of the Royal Sussex Hospital and, despite the rest of the hospital being like a building site, I had a view of the sea. I'd chosen the hospital because it felt close to home, even though Brighton barely felt like home, my having only been there a couple of years. I wanted to have my baby as close as possible to our seafront flat. But it wasn't really home, not yet. I felt isolated and dislocated. My family were a five-hour car journey away (on a good day), or a four-hour train ride. I had a few friends in Brighton, but no one I really shared a history with. No one who really knew me.

From the delivery room I could see the clouds brewing over the sea. We get sea frets all the time on the south coast – sharp squalls and gusts, out of nowhere. The storms were starting to come in at night that autumn, too. Ian and I would sit by the window in our flat and watch them on the sea. The morning after the big storms, the air stank of seaweed and the promenade was covered in stones from the beach, raised into mounds like eerie cairns. The sea saying, I've been here, and here, and here.

Did I feel the depression coming? Did I sense it on the wind, like a sailor catching a whiff of bad weather? An itching scar, tuned into meteorological electrics? Yet I had no scar. I had no war wounds. Save a few heartbreaks, I'd lived a life of good mental health.

Childbirth was a rude awakening, yet it started gently. When I was five days overdue my midwife – my lovely regular midwife – gave me the most mellow, tender sweep. 'I can feel the baby's hair,' she said. I was thrilled. Awed. The creature was coming. And it had … hair.

A few hours later, when my contractions started, I ran a bubble bath and drank a glass of red wine in it to give myself a little send off. Then we headed to the hospital.

Before I go on, I want to say that most of the midwives we saw were wonderful (especially once we got home, and we got a visit every day for a week). They were experienced, kind and professional. But at the hospital, my luck was out.

The hospital was where everything changed. The midwife who met us there was brisk and cold. The first thing she wanted to do was send me home. I said that my contractions were speeding up at a frightening pace and felt ferocious. I'd struggled to get out of the taxi. I knew what I was feeling, knew my body was bucking, and the birth was coming on thick and fast. She said she'd examine me. She spoke to me so disrespectfully, I was almost in tears before her fingers were inside. I was assaulted by a boy on the top deck of a bus when I was thirteen and this felt similar. Her fingers rough and mean; her own agenda to fulfil. It was so upsetting. Compared to the sweep I'd had, it was horrid. It felt like her fingernail cut into me at one point. It made me yelp. I lost all rights to my body in that moment. I lost all autonomy. I didn't know I could say no. I didn't know I could ask for better. I had no idea.

I could have said no as soon as I got the bad vibes from her.

I could have said NO.

And I didn't know.

These are choices. You can say no to anything. So few women know this, while we're organising our Spotify playlists, or imagining that tranquil water birth, or packing our cutest hospital bags. We don't know that if things start to feel uncomfortable or inappropriate, we can refuse our consent. We can ask for other options. We don't have to be such good girls. But maybe by the time we get to giving birth we're feeling so stupid and useless and needy that we have no fight.

After the examination, the midwife said: 'You're only a centimetre dilated. Are you disappointed?' I felt as though she was patronising me. We agreed to go home.

But then I went for a wee on my way out. And during that wee, I bled.

I have no proof, but I'm pretty sure that rough exam was the reason I started bleeding. From that point on, the water birth I'd wanted was out of the question. Once you bleed it's classed as a haemorrhage. I would have to stay in hospital, and I would have to have a cannula inserted into my hand. No fun for a needle-phobe. The cannulas on maternity wards are pretty industrial. (They have to be, for the amount you might potentially bleed.) The midwife I was assigned for my delivery was the opposite of the first – in that she was a nervous wreck. She was also uncommunicative. It took her seven tries – *seven* – to get a cannula the size of a speargun into my hand. I was already spinning out. My contractions were coming so fast that I didn't have time to eat a chocolate brazil between them. (I kept getting halfway and spitting the half-chewed nut out, scared of choking; even more scared of not sucking on the delicious gas and air in time.) I dilated five centimetres in half an hour. I would not lie down. I wanted to stand up. To stomp. To bellow. I was like a marauding ox. I pulled out the cannula, spraying blood everywhere. I can't remember how many goes it took the midwife to get it back in that time. Suddenly, I was having the opposite birth to what I wanted. I was surrounded by machines, wires and needles coming out of me, with a woman whose nervousness was making me nervous.

And where was Ian? He'd taken blood from me for a test during the pregnancy and it had been smooth and painless.

Surely he could get a cannula in, even a whopper? I was feeling abandoned and betrayed, but professional courtesy had got the better of him. Ian was obsessively watching the machines as the baby's heart decelerated – once, twice, three times. We've talked about this lots. I suppose I thought he would step in more, but he was in his own private hell – trapped between his professional knowledge and being a new father in a dangerous environment, where things were going wrong. He disengaged. Clinical detachment. Like a war photographer who frames a dying soldier in his viewfinder, he'd been conditioned to distance his feelings in certain environments in order to focus on the job. How else to cope? I knew how many suicidal patients he regularly talked 'down off the ledge' as a GP. I knew how many people he'd seen die when he'd worked in hospitals. Dead children, dead babies. The places the medical dramas on TV don't dare to go. The two brothers aged five and seven, dead from a house fire, laid out side by side, was the sight that haunted him the most.

I was furious at him for years for leaving me to the mercy of that midwife in that room, but I'm not furious now. He is an excellent doctor. He goes above and beyond. People who hate or fear doctors ask for him specially, because they feel like they can trust him. His kindness and calmness are two of the things I fell in love with. He has become what medicine has made him: the profession that first relies on people's humanity, and then on their detachment.

But it did mean I was left emotionally alone to deal with something I couldn't begin to fathom. There was no one to advocate for me. Things got worse. My midwife didn't believe me when I said my gas and air tank had run out. She insisted she'd checked it. She thought I was a demanding diva, I could tell. She told me off for sucking on the gas and air too much. 'I said only when you're having a contraction!' she yelled at one point. I was in pain, constant pain, I couldn't distinguish between the contractions. They tried an epidural. It failed. The anaesthetist pulled it out and said to Ian: 'It's bleeding – does she have a clotting disorder?' I don't. Ian said no, not that we knew of. At that point it was looking like I might need a c-section under general anaesthetic. Then, the real kicker: my midwife didn't know my son's head was crowning. Which was – spectacularly – just after the gas and air had run out. By this point I was roaring so insistently that a registrar came running in to ask, 'Why is she making that noise?' I'll tell you why 'she' was making 'that' noise: she thought she was fucking dying, and nobody was looking after her.

This all happened between 10 p.m. and 1 a.m. When I first held my son I noticed that we both had blood under our nails, like we'd clawed our way out of something. Little wonder, afterwards, that I had a deep tear on the posterior wall of my vagina and a grazed labia (new band name, anyone?). But it wasn't over. Almost as traumatic as the birth itself were the stitches.

Here are some words you don't want to hear when someone is between your legs, holding a needle and thread aimed at your vagina: 'Should I put a stitch here or here, do you think?'

This was how I found myself, with the same midwife, an hour after the birth. I was in a crazy daze, high on gas and air (which had eventually been replenished – thanks for nothing), trying to grapple with the fact that the midwife had called in someone more experienced to guide her through it. In one way it was perhaps good she was asking the question.

But there was no acknowledgement that this might be absolutely fucking terrifying for me. And it was, absolutely fucking terrifying.

As they discussed my stitches ('It's really hard to see where to put the needle because there's *so much blood* … See what I mean?') I lay there mute, in stirrups, feeling very much like I was in the film *Saw*, where you have to do some hideous mutilating challenge to get out of the room.

I felt like a failure for tearing. Like my vagina was sub-standard somehow. We talk about 'no stitches' like a badge of honour. We pit ourselves against each other like this, as women. *I had my baby in an hour with no stitches!* Is this a woman reassuring herself that she is an adept woman? It's a competitiveness that starts with our periods (*Have you started yet?*) and continues through childrearing (*Where's your baby? Is it as clever/heavy as mine?*). Who puts that on us? I don't think women put it on themselves. I think it's pressed upon us to keep us down. I appreciate that going into something with a positive attitude can affect the outcome, but I also feel as though I was brainwashed into having false expectations. I thought I almost certainly wouldn't tear, when in fact tearing was the most likely thing to happen. According to a study in the *British Journal of Gynaecology*, 85 per cent of women suffer some form of tear during their first vaginal birth. That's a lot of women getting injured! Not only that, but the number of women suffering severe third- and fourth-degree tears (from vagina to anus) tripled from 2 per cent to 6 per cent between 2000 and 2012. The rise has been put down to tears being better diagnosed, but also to women having babies later in life, and bigger babies at that.

And so I wanted to tear and share (sorry), because in

terms of that initial time period, those injuries were as affecting as meeting my baby. And, once I started talking to people about it, the stories flooded in (birth stories in general seem to do this – women hold back, but the stories are there, waiting, like dammed water).

One friend had her labia accidentally stitched together and had to go back, be cut apart and re-stitched correctly. Another friend's c-section scar was rotting and fungal. *They're worth it!* people say. The babies, not the women.

Things go wrong in medicine because it's human beings practising the medicine, I understand that. I also know the NHS suffers from chronic underfunding. If fingers are pointed, it should be at governments. But it strikes me that the injuries and repairs women receive during and after childbirth are talked about even less than childbirth itself. So much so that I didn't even think about them when I was writing my birth plan. All I could think of was another friend's mum who, after giving birth in the 1970s, was brought a cigarette, an ashtray and a box of matches on a trolley. I wanted that kind of afterbirth. Hell, I was so out of it that I forgot to ask to see the placenta (something I *had* been looking forward to). Ian didn't even take a photo! He was so engrossed in the baby. I'm still pretty pissed off about that.

Pregnancy was a time when I shared my body with someone else, but I still felt like a sealed unit. During the birth, I felt like a tin can hacked apart by a knife. For weeks afterwards I was convinced I had a womb infection, that something had got in, such was my feeling of wide-open vulnerability. Early in pregnancy, a friend gave me a book called *The Orgasmic Birth*. Optimistic? Ludicrous! Also: no pressure! I appreciated her intention, though – to remind me that my vagina was more than an escape chute for a tiny human. And I think this is what concerned me most about the stitching. This afterthought, this add-on, this potential botch-job, would determine part of my identity – my sex life – for the rest of my life. If men birthed babies, every delivery unit would have a skilled team of plastic surgeons on call for instant penis repair. Hell, there would be some kind of Nobel Prize for Penis Repair. But women? Nah. Look at the baby, they say – look at the baby! In a sort of 'watch-the-birdy' kind of way. Doesn't it all just melt into insignificance when you see your beautiful baby? The subtext being that it should, if you are not a selfish creature; if you are worthy of mother-hood. Well, I love my baby, but I also love my vagina, and myself. If that makes me a bad mother, so be it. And when I got home and the drugs wore off and I settled into that wild mix of bliss and dread that would colour the next few months, I found I was angry. Livid. That there had been no trust established. Not enough anaesthetic. That even though I pride myself on being assertive, in those stirrups I hadn't spoken up. I wonder how much of this rage, this disappoint-ment, contributed towards the PND. How much I had to bed it down inside me and push, push, push, down instead of out – until it was a roiling mass in my guts, waiting to blow.

I am aware that I write this as a white woman. According to a 2019 report published by the National Perinatal Epide-miology Unit, *MBRRACE-UK* (*Mothers and Babies: Reducing Risk through Audits and Confidential Enquiries Across the UK*), black women in the UK are five (*five!*) times more likely to die during pregnancy and after childbirth than their white counterparts, even though they account for just 4 per cent of those giving birth. For women of mixed ethnicity the risk is threefold; for Asian women, it's double. A report by the Washington Center for Equitable Growth in 2017 showed that black women feel as though they are not listened to with as much empathy and belief as white women during childbirth. They are not taken seriously when they say there is a problem or they feel in pain. Black women have to fight the stereotype that they are angry and aggressive, drama queens, overreacting. Their pain is not taken seriously. They are dismissed as being merely disruptive. And they die because of this. As a white woman I might have been fearful of being seen as troublesome, but I didn't have it any harder because of the colour of my skin.

The mental health of black women is often worse in early motherhood, too. In her book *I Am Not Your Baby Mother: What it's like to be a black British mother*, Candice Brathwaite writes of her own exhaustion and isolation after the birth of her daughter: 'NHS Digital data shows that detention rates under the Mental Health Act during 2017–18 were four times higher for people in the "Black" or "Black British" group than those in the "White" group.'

There are huge conversations that need to be had around childbirth to make it safer for all women. The charity Birthrights states that all women have the right to a safe and positive birth experience, which includes being treated with dignity and respect, and access to pain relief. For something so common, childbirth is too frequently unnecessarily damaging. Too many women are going home from hospital *injured*. I think it's important to use that word. Because these are injuries. They are not inevitable, nor are they badges of honour. They shouldn't be the norm. Women should be informed of the realistic dangers and risks, instead of told that childbirth will be an oxytocin-filled breeze. They should be offered a c-section as an equally accessible option from the start, rather than something to fall back on if they somehow 'fail' to pursue a vaginal delivery for whatever reason. There are two ways to give birth: it isn't the 'natural' way and the 'posh, cowardly' way. You can give birth vaginally or via caesarean section. Let's empower women to make a true choice themselves, rather than feel like they're asking for something that is not reasonable or natural. Natural is a weasel word, and in this context it's deliberately intended to shame women and make them feel disconnected from their body and baby. Well, I drank the 'natural' Kool Aid, and my 'natural' vaginal delivery made me feel utterly disconnected from my body and my baby. Having an operation without anaesthetic is 'natural'. Dying from measles is 'natural'. You know what? Fuck natural. When it hurts people, fuck it.

'Women have to fight to be heard and then are very easily labelled as "difficult",' perinatal psychiatrist Dr Rebecca Moore says. 'I really encourage them to be difficult! If they want a second opinion, or don't click with the midwife, or want someone in the room to introduce themselves ... But most people find it hard to do that, and of course you're going to find it hard to do that if you're in the middle of labour.'

Dr Moore advises women to plan more than their ideal birth – to plan for the ensuing weeks and months, too. 'Plan your social network, your sleep, etc. These are things you can control; birth you can't. I'm not saying you can't have preferences, but you fill in this mythical plan with the expectation that this is how it's going to be. Then it's not – and that is soul-destroying.'

It was soul-destroying for me. And it was just the start.

Something else was born that day. An anxiety. How can I cope with this love, this job, this worry? I was overwhelmed, and sleep deprivation hadn't even got a grip of me yet. I thought childbirth would be the top of the mountain. But it was a fake summit. There was another summit, the kind that comes into view only when you reach the first – except I couldn't see it yet, because it was shrouded by mist, and yet more mystery.

Pregnant Princess;
Postnatal Pauper

During pregnancy, women are showered with attention – and not always the good kind. Once the baby is born, however, it's as though the mother doesn't exist. When I was arguing for a c-section for the birth of my second baby in 2020, I was shocked to hear the surgeon say there was nothing in my birth notes 'to indicate a traumatic birth'. What? Had they swopped my notes or something? Was this gaslighting at an institutional level? Maybe that midwife was as bad at taking notes as she was at delivering babies. Or maybe she thought I was okay throughout it all. Who knows. All I know is: my voice was absent from those notes. I'm sure they got down the baby's weight somewhere, same as they got down his other measurements every step of the way. But my health and wellbeing were left out of the records.

In her book *Constellations*, Sinead Gleeson describes caring for a newborn as being 'static but non-stop'. It is exactly that. A place of paradoxes. Of night and day. Dark and light. Exhaustion and high alert. You feel simultaneously destroyed and reborn.

The afternoon after the birth, I went for a long walk

along the seafront. Ian pushed our son in the buggy and I walked behind. I don't think I was in pain beyond my stitches and grazes, but now I wonder, What the hell was I thinking? I was determined not to be 'beaten' by it. I do remember being scared to tell my parents and sister that I'd had stitches because my sister hadn't had them in either of her deliveries and I felt as though – I know how stupid this sounds – I'd somehow not done well enough. Despite the fact I had no real control over the elasticity of my vaginal wall. And my sister is the loveliest, most generous person in the world. Where did that feeling come from? Was it the proud little swot in me? Childish sibling rivalry? Or was I just realising that the fronting – the separation of the truth of myself, my experience and feelings from the fiction I felt I had to portray – might have to be presented to my family, too? People who had known me all my life? Because that's what started happening.

In some ways it was easy. My family and oldest friends lived far away, up in Manchester. It was relatively easy to fob them off and say I was tired and could only text, as the weeks went on and I withdrew further and further. But of course this was one of the main problems: I was very isolated. We were isolated. Ian's family and old pals were far away, too, in Wales. And we had no one around we felt we could ask for help (the 'I'm at my worst, I haven't washed for two days, please don't talk to me' kind of help). And we felt like we shouldn't have to ask for help anyway. This was parenthood. People did it all the time!

As Ian and I tried to get a routine in place, my physical injuries started to grate. The Grazed Labia, like a true unsigned band, was making a resounding encore most nights. I bought ordinary sanitary pads by mistake, which stuck to the wounds, and peeling them off was a howlingly painful feat. A major problem was the stitches. They just didn't feel right. I couldn't sit down. After a few days of agony, I showed the midwife who came to visit.

'Oh my goodness,' she said, inspecting my battered vulva. 'Someone has decided to be very mean to you.'

'What do you mean?' I said.

'Well, they've left a huge knot on the end.'

That was why I couldn't sit down.

She snipped it off for me. My relief was instant. And momentary.

My abdomen was not vacated. It was not empty. Where there was once a baby there was a knot of anxiety the size of a football. I spent most of the first few weeks asking Ian to pass me things, as I sat or lay down, trapped under a baby. Sandwiches, drinks, the remote control, my phone … I was fearful of reaching for anything lest I disturb the sleeping/feeding babe. I thought I couldn't put a newborn down very often. After a month or so, I became adept at doing everything with one hand, including typing, going to the toilet, and eating a full English breakfast. 'Looking after you is looking after him,' a midwife said. I repeated this to myself often, usually as I was justifying my tenth biscuit. Sugar was my new best friend. Sugar and every terrible overseas property programme on daytime TV. And that show about Australian Border Control, where they find snakes and drugs in people's hats and laptops.

Around this time I have a recurring nightmare where I keep trying to leave the house and every time I get near the door I am detained for another thirty minutes, eternally trapped in a cycle of forgetting things, feeding, winding, and changing nappies. Then I will realise this is not a nightmare; this is real life. The sound of the baby crying makes me panic. It's the strangest thing. It transcends all reason and logic. It's almost as though the sound affects me at a cellular level. My whole body vibrates with the baby's cries and I transform, Hulk-like, into a gibbering, frothing, single-minded wreck, abandoning baskets of shopping in supermarkets and running through town towards home with the buggy, talking in a loud soothing voice so as not to look like a Bad Mother, or someone who has stolen a baby.

They say it takes a village to raise a child for a reason. I actually think caring for a tiny baby is a three-person job. You need one person to be actually caring for the baby, one to be tidying up and preparing meals, and one to be resting. I just don't see how you can do it with fewer people without at least one of them going mad. And both of us went mad, Ian and me. Ian suffered OCD as an adolescent and now, with the sleeplessness and stress, aspects of it started to resurge as my depression took a hold.

I'd like to say the midwife snipping off that knot was where the physical discomfort ended at least. But my son came out with a huge haematoma, like a little Conehead, likely caused during the fast birth as he knocked and scraped his head against one of my pelvic bones. It injured us both, and I went on to have hip pain for two years. My hips hurt every night – sometimes so much I cried, maxed out on painkillers, unable to get comfortable, told by my GP it was 'normal' to have pain for 'about a year' after childbirth. I couldn't lie on my side in bed. I couldn't take any decent painkillers because I was breastfeeding. This pain was another contributing factor, I am sure, of the continued slow chipping away at me; the disintegration I was undergoing that was sapping my strength and leaving me increasingly vulnerable. My son's haematoma took only a little longer than my hip pain to dissipate. It has only just calcified within his growing skull, and is something you'd know was there only if you knew to feel for it. I often kiss it.

People say that with postnatal depression you feel numb, nothing, towards the baby. But I didn't feel that way. I had an instant urge to protect him, but it wasn't what I'd call bonding. (The only thing I was bonding to was the wrong kind of maternity pad. Ouch.) Trouble was, I felt so far away from my usual 'normal', I didn't know where my feelings were. How could I know what was wrong with me? Or what this all meant?

I called him 'the baby' instead of his name for the first six months or so. When I pushed the buggy down the street, I stood to one side of it, pushing with one hand. Partly to keep my sore back straighter, but I can't help but read the metaphor between the lines: I literally couldn't get behind the job of motherhood. I was one foot in, one foot out.

And then there was the sleep deprivation. My son was a bad sleeper from the start. There are not even words to describe the level of tiredness I experienced. 'Bone-tired' is the closest I can get, but my bones felt like they'd dissolved – along with my frontal lobe. There is a reason sleep deprivation is used as torture. I was so tired I kept repeating sentences. I was so tired I kept repeating sentences. At night, in bed, I got flashes of bright white behind my eyes – bursts of adrenaline, I learned – the split second the baby started crying.

Every time the baby went to sleep I felt the way I did when I'd finished a novel. A hyper sense of achievement.

I was manic with joy and a sudden sense of my own use-lessness. Emptied out. Hollow. Evolved to a sort of bitter nirvana. Unsure what to do with myself. The urge to go on a bender was strong. And then that anxiety had nowhere to go. But the real killer was the guilt. Because this was meant to be some kind of golden age of life. I was meant to feel lucky, and grateful, and fulfilled. Complete. My grandma kept saying it to me: 'Well, Emma, now you have everything you ever wanted.' I want to cry down the phone every time she says it. I want to say:

I have no sleep, Gran.

I'm a pit of anxiety.

My relationship is almost in pieces.

I think my career is over.

My body hurts in fifty places and there's nothing I can do about it and I'm terrified I'm broken for ever.

But she is ninety years old and I don't want to upset or disappoint her. So instead I do what I do with the rest of my family and friends: I say I'm fine. It becomes like a well-worn prayer, the 'I'm fine' mantra. But I wasn't feeling complete. I was fragmenting into a million pieces, and I was starting to blow away.

When the baby is a month old, I go to meet two friends at the Grand Hotel on the seafront for afternoon tea. Leaving the house is, every time, like one of those bad dreams where you're wading through treacle and late for something important, like a flight. I pack up the buggy with endless gubbins and make it out onto the street. The hotel is only a twenty-minute walk from my flat but I'm already late. One thing I am thankful for though: the baby is sleeping. I feel pleased that I have managed to feed him before we set out, so he might sleep now for an hour at least and give me some time to socialise. When I get to the hotel, I realise the table my friends have been seated at is in the conservatory, where the gaps between the tables are too narrow for a buggy. I feel the panic start to rise in my throat.

Years earlier, I'd watched my sister run out of restaurants, abandoning family meals, to take my crying baby nephew outside. She'd sit with him in the car, breastfeeding, vowing to go without food herself – rather that than the stress of feeling like her baby was ruining someone else's dining experience. I'll admit I'd thought it was a bit ridiculous. Now, I feel the exact same urge. The same lack of appetite. The same bile-force of discomfort.

At the Grand, I smile meekly at my friends at their table in the civilised conservatory. The chinaware and silver clinks. There are trolleys of dainty cakes being wheeled around. It is early December and the hotel has been done up for Christmas. My friends have been waiting for me to order and are sharing a pot of tea.

I manage to squeeze the buggy through the tables to them, apologising constantly, trying not to think that people are dismayed or annoyed to see a baby coming into their midst.

I greet my friends, shrug off my jacket and wonder whether to order a glass of prosecco. God, I miss going out.

But whether it's the change in temperature, or the cessation of motion, or just the sense of me relaxing, the baby wakes as soon as I sit down. I stare at him, willing him not to wail. *Don't wail don't wail don't wail, please.*

He wails.

My friends try to talk to me. They ask me how I am. They

are not bothered by the wailing. Maybe no one is bothered by the wailing.

I am bothered by the wailing. I can't concentrate. I try and answer their question. How am I? How *am* I?

Wail wail.

It is impossible.

The waiter comes to take our order.

It is too late. I am fully engaged in panic mode. My heart pounds. I panic. Here we are, ruining all these people's afternoon teas!

'I'm sorry,' I say, getting up. I manoeuvre the buggy out again, knocking the corners of tables as I pass – sorry, so sorry – just trying to get out of the room, out of earshot.

I push the buggy into the accessible toilet. I pull the baby out of the buggy and start to breastfeed. He goes quiet. I exhale. My phone vibrates. It is one of my friends. 'Are you okay?'

Yes, I reply. Five minutes. Sorry, you go ahead and order.

But I sit in there longer than five minutes. I feed him and then I realise that I am afraid. I do not want to go back into the restaurant. I feel very far away from all of those people, including my friends. I want to go home. Except the urge is simpler than that; less positive and comforting. I want to hide.

I look around the toilet. Even in the Grand Hotel, breastfeeding in a toilet is a fairly grim affair. I am far from mastering breastfeeding confidently in public – and this just compounds my feelings of shame, failure and the need to run away to a secret dark place where I can do my baby business in private. The NCT classes I attended forced upon me a huge pressure to breastfeed. But it was amazing how few places there were to breastfeed in comfort and confidence. If they're going to pressure us, maybe at least back it up with more facilities? Or make women feel safer getting their tits out? There is propaganda everywhere featuring the word 'natural', and a resulting sense of failure for those who don't breastfeed, or didn't have a vaginal delivery, as difficult as these things so often are. Again, it's the weaselly 'natural' chat. But what if the natural was trying to tame me and box me up? Put me somewhere society could keep an eye on me and see another obedient daughter playing at being another obedient mother. But I was too bewildered to have such complex thoughts back then, in that toilet. I was shattered. I was floundering.

I put the baby back in the buggy and sneak back into the lobby and out of the main doors. I send my bewildered friends apologetic text messages from the road as I run, crying.

'Are you really okay?' they text.

'Yes, fine!' I insist. My mantra. My living lie. 'Just getting used to breastfeeding!'

They didn't press it. Were they embarrassed in their own way? Did the taboos for women stretch in every direction, making us all afraid to talk, to ask, to cry, to scream?

Tits and Tropes

'Don't write about breastfeeding, whatever you do!' Katie warned me.

'Why?' I said. 'It's fucking awful! I have so much to say!'

'No,' she said, 'no no no no no.'

'But why?'

'Because, Emma, BEWARE THE TROPES OF THE NEW MOTHER.'

She's right, of course. Katie is a seer and a soothsayer. Brutally honest is another way of putting it. Breastfeeding is a killer. I decided to do it because somehow the idea of pumping my breasts seemed more depressing. Too bovine. But I soon realised how hard breastfeeding is.

I hate the conspiracy of silence – yet another! – around the reality of breastfeeding. No one tells you that initially your baby will be starving (they will survive, but they will be starving) in the time between your colostrum running out and your milk coming in, and that during this time, nothing will soothe them, and you will be beside yourself. The first night, the baby screamed and screamed – for hours. Ian carried him around the room while I lay in bed, anguished. I thought he was in agony. I was pretty sure he'd be traumatised. We were already doing it wrong! We were already fucking him up!

Decades later, in therapy, his shrink would tell him that the reason he hates this time of night, the reason he cannot get to sleep, the reason he hates breasts, and women, and himself, is because his mother had no food for him the first night of his life. Ian eventually rocked him to sleep and settled him. I'll never forget the words Ian used as he laid him in the co-sleeper. I'd never heard him say those words before, but he's said them plenty since, and I have adopted them myself when talking to our son: 'There we are,' he said as he laid the exhausted baby down, dummy in (he never took a dummy after that first night), swaddled in a muslin covered in blue stars. The baby was asleep.

I felt my chest relax. The breath push out of me. I do not breathe right whenever my baby is upset, which means I often do not breathe right because babies are often upset. If only I had known I could have given him a bottle of formula and we all would have settled. I didn't feel as though that was in my arsenal. I *had* to do it all by breast. I had to. That was the rule. The other options, as with childbirth, had been presented to me as back-ups, as cop-outs. 'You've just got to keep the faith,' one midwife told me. But there is a reason I am not religious. I understand that they don't want the baby to be confused by a bottle when they haven't got used to a nipple, but some honesty wouldn't go amiss.

'Breast is best,' they say at the NCT classes, on every leaflet; every piece of propaganda. I find myself yelling FOR WHOM? There needs to be a lot more support for women to breastfeed if they choose, and to not breastfeed if they choose. A friend of mine said recently, 'Where are all the bottle-feeding counsellors?' Which is a good point.

Colostrum (the first few days of breastmilk) has some

clear benefits – it has antibodies and is also a mild laxative that helps the baby's bowels get moving and pass meconium – but I think the science is out on whether breastmilk after that is better than formula. Plus, regardless of the science, there are two people in the equation, not one. There is a mother as well as a baby. A mother who is often exhausted, confused, lost and usually in some kind of pain or discomfort. Is this the best we can expect? Really?

My milk finally came in a few days after the birth. Boy oh boy, did it. I remember standing in front of the mirror, amazed at my huge, conical, dripping breasts. 'Engorged' is an ugly, sexy word. But as I started to feed my baby, it was hard to know how much he was getting. I wished for see-through breasts so I could see how much was in there. Then I realised what I was wishing for. I was wishing to be a dairy farm.

Breastfeeding was not 'best' for me. Far from it. It was fucking dreadful for me. I got mastitis, which came on as shivers in the night. I couldn't bear for the duvet to touch my nipples. Ian took my temperature. 'You have a fever,' he said. I thought I had a womb infection after the birth had left me feeling so vulnerable and cracked open. But then I felt gristly lumps in my left breast. Blocked ducts, trapped milk. Rotting inside me. The pain was terrible. I took painkillers – bullshit paracetamol that has never touched the sides but is all mothers are allowed – and didn't feel any improvement. The next day I went and got antibiotics. The antibiotics gave me thrush – that lovely little chaser.

I start calling my left boob 'Bad Boob'. As well as the mastitis, this is the boob that leaks more, it is the boob that sprays unevenly. It has caught the baby out a few times, in his eye. (But then again he's pissed in his own mouth on the changing mat, so he's got bigger issues.)

Breastfeeding didn't bond me to my baby. It made me hate my baby. Everywhere I turned, there it was, his mouth, yawning before me like an abyss: the terrible, insatiable need of him. I started to see the ridged, red chasm of his mouth as THE ENEMY. I became a contortionist. I was so desperate to quieten him, I hurt my back by raising my leg a little off the floor to tilt him at the right angle. I pulled a neck muscle craning my neck to kiss him while he was feeding.

'Mother Nature is a misogynist,' I told my friend Jenn. 'There's no other explanation. I'm meant to feel all fuzzy and fulfilled. I feel the opposite.'

Jenn agrees. Jenn is a big reader. She says, 'When I was a teenager I never really understood what D. H. Lawrence was going on about when he wrote of the "bitter, bone-deep enmity" between men and women. Now I know it's about childrearing.'

Yep. Because Ian isn't going through this, is he? And I do hate him for that. I know I shouldn't, but I do. I'm starting to. My bones are starting to turn against him.

But more than anything, breastfeeding becomes just one of many things I hate myself for hating. I hate the fact I can't get on with my work. I hate the fact I keep eating entire packs of biscuits just to not feel tired. I hate the fact that most of my shoes don't fit and probably never will again. I hate the way that there's such pressure to breastfeed and yet there's nowhere clean and private to do it anywhere in town. I hate the way I am not fierce enough to just get my tits out and think *fuckit*. I hate all this fear and guilt and fretfulness that has sprung out of nowhere. What else? I hate my telescopic nipples, my mashed fanny, and the fact that there is no running away from any of this. Quite the opposite: I am *inside* the problem.

D. H. Lawrence might have been right, because I'm directing more and more of these dark feelings towards Ian. I hate the way he doesn't have to stop at a few glasses of wine if he doesn't want to. How he can go out for the whole day without planning it. How he sleeps deeply because he can still completely shut down without a small part of his brain left on, even when he's asleep, poised to detect a stir amongst the blankets in the crib, or the tiniest tentacle of a wail. How his body is not still a stranger to him, after months now of mystery, of amazement, of surrender. I am at my lowest and darkest. I haven't been to these depths in myself since I was heartbroken aged twenty-two. That's fifteen years ago.

One night, Ian stays out a bit later than agreed at the pub and when he gets back I am ready to stab him. I'VE BEEN DOING ALL THIS ON MY OWN FOR FUCKING HOURS, I scream, deranged. My back hurts from the baby wanting to be constantly walked up and down or else he won't go to sleep. I feel like the most miserable bagpipe player, pacing, plodding, with a swaddled bag on my shoulder.

Ian is worried, really worried then. He suggests I reach out to my family. But my family are miles away. And I like to be self-sufficient. But he is right. I have never been less self-sufficient. I am flailing, goddammit. I send a few messages. The next day he goes out and buys a Christmas tree. A white twinkling pre-lit one. It changes the room, and my mood. Also – what I don't say, what I maybe don't even realise, but I realise now – is that *we* used to go out together. Ian and I. We loved pubs. We loved meals out. They were a joy. They were a big foundation stone for our relationship. Gone, all gone.

A few afternoons later, the door buzzer goes. I am agitated by this – I don't like unexpected guests, and I look like shit, and I feel like shit, and—

I answer.

It is my new friend Alex, from the NCT course. She is French-Canadian and full of joie de vivre. She calls me 'buddy'. She comes in with her buggy and her baby and several bags. In the bags are special gifts, salt and flour, so I can make salt-dough impressions of the baby's feet. She also brings some sausages, kale and parsnip mash because 'they were on offer'. She sits next to the Christmas tree. I tell her she is like a Magus. One of the Three Wise (Wo)men. She shakes off the compliment because it's just what she does.

She stays an hour and then she leaves. I watch her jiggle into the lift and something shifts inside of me. Something is punctured.

I take the salt and flour up to my parents' house the following week. I mix the dough, squish the baby's feet in, and bake three little hard patties of his feet. It's a good thing to do. It stills the world and my worries for a moment – gathers everything that's spinning into a solid point in time, captured and cast. I Facetime Alex to thank her, and our babies press hands on the laptop screen.

Alex is a good mother. Not just of her baby, but of her friends. You don't have to have kids to be maternal. You can mother everyone around you, even yourself. I have always believed that. A good woman has reminded me. I tell breastfeeding and Mother Nature that I am introducing a three-strikes-and-you're-out rule and, after the mastitis and the thrush, she has one strike left. Then I'm putting the baby on formula. I apply a magic lanolin cream after every feed. I'll never be a natural, but it's a bit more bearable for a few months. I still feel shaky, though. Still feel quite unlike myself. Like I am uprooted and ragged. Like I am adrift and small.

But when Alex calls and asks me how I am, I can't admit my real feelings. How scared I am, how tired I am, how lonely I am, how low I am. How much I hate it all. I can't tell this lovely, kind, normal woman the truth. So I do what I am so good at now: I lie.

Then Mother Nature throws another curveball. The baby gets teeth. At sixteen weeks. He starts biting me. I get scabs on my nipples and have to breastfeed through the scabs. (This is when I start doing silent screams, letting my head fall back and opening my mouth wide – blowing air and all my anger at the ceiling, while he sucks on, regardless. At least I hope he is regardless.) One time, he draws blood in a café. I howl. This is above and beyond. I don't know it's teeth at first, though. Who else's baby had teeth at sixteen weeks? No one's! I thought it was just normal to get bitten, and bleed, and scab over, and go through it again. (There is a lot I am accepting as 'normal' by this point.) I mean, it's horrific. I am soaking breast pads with blood, like they're sanitary pads. My nipples are bleeding so much I feel like I need a SWAT team on stand-by to come in and rescue me whenever he bites. I fantasise about them storming through the windows and whisking me away from danger, Sigourney Weaver at the helm, taking no shit. *Get her out of there!* She'd bundle me up in a helicopter and we'd fly to the other side of the world, taking my nipples to safety.

But no one gets me out of there. Someone does give me some important information, though. A cranial osteopath I go and see, to show her the baby's haematoma, is examining him when I casually mention the fact that breastfeeding is making me bleed. She looks at me oddly.

'Bleed? How much?'

'Oh, lots. But that's not the worst of it really. Don't get me started on my hips ...'

She narrows her eyes. 'He's sixteen weeks?' she says.

'Yes,' I reply.

She opens his mouth.

'Do you think his teeth might be coming?' I ask.

'No,' she says, 'it would be very early for that. When they get teeth they get – oh!' She jumps. Pulls his lip down to show me his gum, which is seeded with strips of pale white. 'They get things that look like little grains of rice in their gums. Just like that.'

She closes his mouth and looks at me.

'Your baby is teething.'

'Oh. Okay. Wow. Great.'

Teething! At sixteen weeks. I want a word with the Tooth Fairy or whoever is in charge of this shit.

I remember when I was pregnant hearing horror stories that some babies came out with full sets of teeth. As a pregnant woman, amongst pregnant women, I would inhale and shudder at this. A monster-baby with teeth! Arrgh. At the time, this was terrifying. Now, I think: what a total fucking dream. Get the teething out of the way while they're in the womb: SOUNDPROOFED. Brilliant.

Because at sixteen weeks, it was a problem. You can't 'tell off' tiny babies. You can't say *No!* when they bite you, like you can with bigger babies. Tiny babies don't have the ability to store the information and remember it for next time. They don't have the processing facilities. They aren't ready to learn to adapt their behaviour. They just get upset. So I kept going with the breastfeeding for another month. I think I was really without most of my self-respect by this point.

In addition to the physical side of things, I find breastfeeding hard ideologically. It's an unfair division of labour. Plus, other people make me feel uncomfortable for doing it in public. A few of the women from my NCT group have had comments directed towards them when they've been breastfeeding out and about, and I am primed for such an attack. I have lines prepared: *So? This ain't no peep show! It's a restaurant not a strip club, sweetheart!* And: *He's just having his lunch, too, for Chrissakes!* Under the Equality Act 2010 it's illegal to stop a woman breastfeeding anywhere. Anywhere! I feel like this is a law people should know, now it affects me daily. Like the law about giving way to pedestrians crossing a side road, rather than shouting at them for not looking. I can't believe women haven't made more of the breastfeeding-anywhere thing. We all creep around, worried about exposing our nipples and offending a society that charges people to see them. It's not my fault that women's breasts have been commodified and therefore make some people feel sexual/uncomfortable/both.

Part of the reason I stay at home more, part of the reason I don't want to leave the flat is because I feel panicky about feeding him in public. About getting my tits out. It is always a grapple with the shawl. Those shawls! One time I thought I was covered and realised from the top I was but my whole tit was exposed at the back, to a full café. I'd lost too much of my fight and bite to think, *Fuck it*. It was never a smooth manoeuvre. I never got the hang of slings, either.

I wanted an app that could let me know where was good to feed and change a baby. (Can someone design this, please?) The worries swarmed before each trip outside. Would there be somewhere to sit? I needed a comfy seat with the right leg-height so my feet could be flat on the floor. Would I be able to find somewhere meeting these requirements in time when he started bawling? The sound of him crying made me panic, too. I didn't know what he was crying for – I only learned after a month that babies cry when they are tired. (He was also teething.) And sometimes they cry for no reason at all. They just fancy a quick – to use a good old Lancastrian word – skrike. I thought it was always food! The message is FEED FEED FEED. A successful mother is a feeding mother. A successful mother is a mother with a fat baby. It can feel so much easier to stay in your own living room with your top off, watching overseas property programmes and eating sugar.

There's also a lot of misinformation around alcohol and breastfeeding. No one can really investigate it, obviously. Aside from the ethics, there's no real pressure or impetus to. It's only women's lives being restricted, after all. It's all very vague and general, even from the NHS; the official line being the only proven safe amount of alcohol to drink during breastfeeding is nothing. I chat to my paediatrician friend Alex about this. She says that the lethal level for alcohol poisoning is 0.4 per cent alcohol in the blood. Breast milk cannot amplify any alcohol in the blood; it is, at most, the same concentration. So even if you had ingested enough alcohol to kill you, there would be less alcohol in your breast milk than in a non-alcoholic beer. The next time I see her, we have a whisky. While we breastfeed. *But it's a neurotoxin!* the breastfeeding police cry. Sure, and so are exhaust fumes, which you inhale plenty of if you live in a city, or near a road. Modern life is toxic. We don't need to shame women for having the odd drink.

I told myself it was the teeth. It wasn't. It was the inhibition and lack of freedom. The difficulties of breastfeeding added to an already heavy load. I suppose what I'm saying is if a woman is in pain for long enough, and denied sleep for long enough, and at the same time feels as though she has to keep going and put a 'brave' face on, she's going to crack. But I was clueless. I was in the dark, and it was getting darker. It was January, coming into February. I was crying more often. I was shouting more often. When I looked out to sea, the horizon had disappeared. Mists and ghosts were everywhere. I could not find my way home, to anyone, or anything.

I couldn't stop thinking about the notion of demonic possession. It was a notion that had obsessed me years earlier, when I was going through a break-up and living in a big house, which I was often alone in. I kept thinking a demon was coming for me. It's partly because I love horror films – but it's also because for me, mental illness is synonymous with the idea of being hunted and taken over. But it had never been as bad as this before. This time, it was going to consume me. I wonder now how much it was to do with an awareness of misdiagnosis in the past of so many mental illnesses (especially in women and girls) – where people were thought to be possessed by demons or spirits. I think I was becoming aware of something misdiagnosed or undiagnosed in me. Those days when I felt a *blackblackblack* and a *lowlowlow* that I could barely find normal words to describe.

Something was coming, I could feel it. A raging storm of some kind. Did I have the strength to meet it and survive?

Ian and I loved storms. We'd watched them many nights from our balcony, forked lightning flashing the sea water purple. But this one, this one was different. Bigger. Inside the house. It wasn't a fun thrill to be experienced from the safety of inside. It was pulling me out of the window, ripping my hair from my head, filling my mouth with icy air so I couldn't scream for help. The pressure. The low pressure.

Falling. Rising.

Something was coming for me.

Something was coming.

Burning Out

Our flat in Brighton was close to the old burnt-out West Pier. The pier was set on fire in 2003 and is now a dark skeleton, a gothic silhouette on the seascape. It's all the more beautiful for being desolate. Much more pleasant to look at than the working pier. There's a red buoy in the sea that marks its edge, to warn boats and swimmers that there are dangerous pieces of iron submerged just beneath the surface. Pieces of the pier fall away every time there is a storm. In wintertime, starlings roost in what remains of the shabby rafters. At night, the buoy flashes with a red light every five seconds or so. When we first moved in, Ian and I watched it together often as we sat looking out to sea, having a cup of tea or a glass of wine. When the baby was small I watched it alone, up breastfeeding all times of the day and night. I wrote snatches of things down on scraps of paper during this time. I found one of them while I was looking through my old diaries for this book.

> Get up. Is he crying? You heard something, that's why you woke. Must be. Or energy. Sometimes you think you still share a pulse. You wake, he wakes. He wakes, you wake. There is no lonely. No reprieve. You pick up

your socks. Don't put your socks on yet, you'll slip on the floor. These are not your socks. No these are your socks, it's okay. Put your socks on.

I wrote these words during the first few months of being a mother. I don't usually keep a notebook about my life. I note down thoughts for various projects I'm working on in separate A5 journals, but this was on a scrap of paper torn from my weekly planner. It troubled me when I found it. It's a weird little paragraph (why the obsession with socks?) and I don't remember writing it: whether it was day or night; whether I intended to do anything with it, show it to anyone, or merely document my feelings at that point. I have never been much of a diarist. But I had also never been a mother before. All bets were off.

The thing that troubles me the most about these words is not the fact they point to the sleep deprivation, which was already becoming an issue and, I think, the thing that made me the most ill. Nor is it the fact that everyday things were starting to feel alien – even my own socks. No, it's how they show me drifting away from myself, like someone having an out-of-body experience. I do not know the woman who wrote these words, and yet I was her. Now, it seems like the clear beginning of a detachment from a sense of self; an abstraction of my whole life and identity. It also seems a lot like denial: aka the first stage of grief. When I look back and try to remember that person, I don't know her. I go down streets in Brighton, where I still live, streets I remember from when I used to trudge along them, pushing the buggy – and the memories of those days are cold-blooded. I feel as though I'm watching a film about someone else's life rather than remembering my own.

How did I get so far away from myself?

I remember the health visitor coming to see us. She was a nice woman. I tidied up like it was a date, or like I was meeting my mother-in-law. Worse: it was like I was on trial. Guilty until proven innocent. Certainly wanting to seem perfect. I was careful to turn around any books – my own included – that might reference alcohol, smoking or drugs, or any kind of violence or murder or freakiness (i.e. most of my book collection).

There are two great underlying fears for mothers, I think, and these ultimate fears inform every attempt to avoid shame and judgement: your baby is going to die, or (worse, somehow, socially) your baby is going to be taken away. It is from that fearful bedrock that we are frightened, harassed and bullied into conforming. Into being 'kept safe' by and for society, and by 'safe' I mean fearful. Unlikely to bitch or bolt. We suppress our truths.

I wanted to convince the health visitor how perfect I was for the job. It felt more like a job interview than a check-up for my benefit. I think that's the point that strikes me now – it didn't feel like it was for me. I want to laugh at this person now. WTF was I thinking? Why was I trying to be Doris Day? But I was so full of anxiety, so full of the idea that I should have metamorphosed into some kind of flawless new creature. I was so busy trying to look perfect – the model mother and housewife – that I forgot to tell the truth. I didn't really listen to the questions. I wanted her validation, I wanted boxes ticked, and then I wanted her out. I also think I was living in such a flurry – on high alert, on adrenaline – that I was skimming the top of everything without analysing much. So I wasn't labouring over how to lie to her. I was just rushing to get to the next thing my baby might need (he always needed something). I was living at full pelt.

Even though I live in Brighton, a liberal hotspot full of progressives, every single couple I encountered – from the NCT group to Baby bloody Boogie – involved the woman taking time out from her career but not the man. Every woman I know in a het couple gave up her work for at least six months to become a parent. And this was Brighton. Relatively rich. Certainly progressive. It has a lot to do with breastfeeding, but it seems so widespread, and it has repercussions. The men are 'working', so they get priority for sleep. But the women are working too. Long, hard hours. Motherhood is a full-time job. Domestic labour is unrecognised, unpaid graft. Cooking, cleaning, washing, childcare – all of these things make a home function, and yet they are seen as just part of life. But it causes problems in terms of financial independence, and feeling empowered and safe. Ian and I still occasionally argue when he talks about how 'he was paying all the bills during this time'. He was earning money because he could, but we were both 'paying the bills'. And arguably, for me, it was working out a *lot* more expensive in terms of my mental health.

The women I knew during my first six months of new motherhood were getting up in the night, every night, with no respite except perhaps half a day at the weekend when their partner 'babysat' so they could have a nap, or a run, or a shower. Not only this, but the mental load – knowing things like how much and when the baby feeds, which clothes fit, when the next jabs are due – falls within women's domain. For a group of people I am sure would all identify as feminists, this is pretty shit. Perhaps as children get older the work is more evenly shared out, but with babies it's the women doing most of the work, more often than not. My brain was getting overloaded with it, and I had nowhere to share, nowhere to download. Combined with the anxiety, it was lethal.

'So many people don't enjoy the first year of motherhood, and that's really sad,' says Sara Campin, founder of the Nourish app, designed to give mothers better mental wellbeing and soothe their frazzled nerves. Sara was inspired to create the app after finding herself 'exhausted and dissatisfied' after the birth of her two children. 'I started thinking, surely I can't be the only mother who's not enjoying this,' she says. 'People were talking more and more about the struggle but no one was saying, "This is how you find more joy in it." With Nourish we want to empower women and teach them ways to be more compassionate to themselves.'

Launched in 2019, Nourish offers bite-sized chunks of coaching every day – from five-minute mindfulness meditations to mini yoga sessions and mood-boosting tips. I use it myself and I love it. I'm sad I didn't have it in 2016. Campin says she has discovered a growing maternal wellbeing community online. 'There are so many barriers for mothers around self-care: time, guilt, it's fluffy, or it's not cool,' she says. 'But taking time out enables you to be a better mum. The app offers lots of different tools, formats and lengths. It's support in your pocket, at your fingertips. It can transform the way you practise self-care. It's about how you soothe yourself.'

Back in 2016 and 2017, there was no space left in my head for me. When I imagined being a mother, I genuinely thought the baby would fit around my life. 'Really, I do the perfect job for motherhood,' I'd raved to friends. 'I can work from home in my pyjamas!' The laugh I want to do now, remembering this – a sort of anguished HAHAHARRRRG-GGGGGG – would take up the entire wordcount of the rest of this book.

My friend Katie is one of the smartest women I know. We've been friends since I was twenty-two. She is elegant and erudite, literary and sophisticated. She sails through any social situation you throw her into, like a swan but with really good jewellery. She doesn't talk; she purrs like Nigella. (I met Nigella Lawson at a book launch once and all I could think was *God, you remind me of Katie*.) Men fall over themselves to talk to her. A male friend I once held a torch for said, after meeting her at a festival: 'I fell a little bit in love with Katie.' 'Yeessss,' I replied wearily (slightly jealously), 'we *all* fall a little bit in love with Katie …'

Katie was a single mum who had her son when she was in her early twenties. I remember saying my stock phrase to her when I was pregnant – *I can work during his naps!* – and her looking at me with a sort of wistful teariness. Like she was sad about something, far off in the distance. Now I know what she was sad about. It was my tragic, soon-to-be-massacred innocence. She said to me, years later, 'Yes, I have to bite my tongue when I hear people about to become parents saying things like that. It just wouldn't do to impose my experience upon their hope. And there is a chance they'll find it different. A very small chance.'

I appreciate her not pissing on my chips.

She told me another thing when I said I was barely replying to emails, never mind getting any writing done. 'Ah,' she said. 'The baby deal-making has begun.'

I asked her what she meant by this.

'Well, shortly after you realise the baby is a time and energy leech (harsh but true), you try and make deals with it. You say, "Okay, baby, I see you. So how about we cut a deal? How about I give you 80 per cent of myself and just keep aside a meagre 20 per cent for me?"

'"*No!*" says the baby. "I want all of you."

'"Okay, okay, I'm sure we can come to some sort of reasonable arrangement," you say. "How about 90/10?"

'"*No!*" says the baby. "ALL OF YOU!"

'"Be reasonable!" you plead. "Would you accept 95 per cent?"

'"Nah-ah." The baby shakes its head. "All. Of. You."

'"Okay, okay," you say, exhausted, defeated. "You can have all of me."

'The baby smiles. "And that bit too," it says.

'"Which bit?"

'"The bit you're hiding behind your back."

'"Goddamn you! How did you spot that?"

'"Hahaha. Don't think you can hide anything from me."

'You hand it over. You hand over every last part of yourself.

'"And that bit there, inside the trapdoor inside your soul."

'"But I didn't even know there was a trapdoor in my soul! That's not fair!"

'"Your special reserves. I want it all. I need it all. You cannot deny me! I AM YOUR CHILD."

'And so you hand that over, too. The parts of you that you didn't even know existed. You are rinsed. Truly spent. This kid has shaken you down. That's the thing with babies. They're all take-take-take.'

Katie tells me all of this with a wry laugh. I laugh too. But I think, *Fuck, my life is over*.

Another close friend of mine, Aimee, has already admitted defeat with her one-year-old. 'Just surrender,' she advises. 'Don't fight it. It's a lot easier when you just surrender.' I find this chilling. But the worst thing is, I can't even tell my oldest, best friends the truth of how I'm feeling. I joke about it. I minimise my thoughts and feelings, I squish myself further and further into a hole.

In Brighton I am in a WhatsApp group of lovely local women who I did the NCT course with – eight of us in total – but they all seem to be getting on with things, and no one has mentioned feeling sad or anxious. We start hanging out with one couple in particular, two doctors called Alex and Simon who are still our great friends. We had bonded in the lift on the way to the first NCT session when we were the only couples to be late: instant kindred spirits. But now I find myself wanting to impress them, as new friends, rather than tell them how hard I am finding things. Similarly, there are two women in my block of flats who had babies within the same month as me, but they seem so calm and chilled. (Now, in retrospect, I wish I'd spoken out, because I'm sure they were finding at least some things hard.)

'There's not an instinct for parenting,' says neuroscientist Dr Jodi Pawluski. 'You still have to figure out how to bath your baby and do all these things. Anyone can be a parent, you just have to be motivated or have the desire. I think it's a primary caregiver thing. Brain changes can occur just as much, perhaps differently due to hormones, but just as much, in primary caregivers that are not biological.'

My brain felt like it was simply disappearing. I am not

good at doing nothing. Of course it's not nothing. It's baby-care. It's everything. It is another paradox: everything and nothing all at once. The mindless repetition of it: nappies, feeding, soothing, changing, nappies, feeding, soothing, changing. I felt like I was losing control of my life, and I didn't know how to take back that control because my usual way would be to write, but I was too tired, and too frightened that my writing meant nothing now, and too scared that everything I wrote felt public somehow, and too damn confused to even begin with a sentence that might be the start of something I could not finish. I had no way to let the words just pour out, which was what I needed to do.

Part of the way I dealt with the anxiety was to become a strategic planner. Someone who gave a running commentary. Someone who said their to-do list out loud, like an automaton. 'Now, we'll go outside.' 'Now, we'll have our lunch.' I said things like this when I was alone with the baby. But I wasn't talking about me and the baby. That wasn't the 'we'. The 'we' was me and the people I needed to be. The people I was detaching into.

In December I realise I have not had more than four hours of straight sleep for over a month. Most nights the baby wakes every hour or so. It is maddening. As the months go on, and the year moves deeper into winter, I gradually get darker inside. I have to start working again – I *want* to start working again. I am a self-employed writer, and it hasn't come easy. But new mothers are not supported, financially or holistically, by the state or system – apart from a small amount I could claim as self-employed.

Ian is overwhelmed too, and exhausted. He is worried he is so tired that he's making bad decisions as a GP. I am becoming a person he doesn't know; a person who screams and shouts and sends spiteful texts. With no extended family nearby, we just have to keep working and not sleeping and feeling like we're doing a shit job of the lot. When I compare myself to other people and other descriptions of motherhood, my pride clouds things. I feel like a loser for not coping. I am baking (I do not bake). I am posting happy pictures. I am doing my best I'M FINE dance all over town. I want to look like a capable person. A modern woman. A successful feminist, having it all her way.

The Weirdest Thing
I've Ever Done in
a Hotel Room

London Book Fair, March 2017. It was one of my first trips out on my own without the baby. I was still breastfeeding and had to drain my breasts every four hours max. I travelled to London on the train to meet my American editor, a dapper New York gent in his seventies who'd edited the likes of Hemingway and Burroughs. We always had a slap-up lunch whenever he was in town.

I went to his hotel in Sloane Square and arrived twenty minutes early so I'd have time to nip to the toilet in the lobby and pump my breasts before meeting him at the entrance. I was petrified of my boobs leaking during lunch. Usually we went to some cool, arty, pastel-hued little Italian place. But when I got to the hotel he was there, waiting in the lobby already.

'Oh hi!' I said, off-guard, gutted.

'Emma!' He was wearing a trilby and tweed coat. I loved this guy. I didn't want to be some lactating loser in front of this guy.

'You're early.'

'Yes,' I said, considering my options for lying. Maybe my brain was too tired for invention, because I just told him the truth.

'I never thought I'd say this to you,' I said, 'but I need to pump my breasts in the loo before lunch.'

He was unfazed. 'Use my room!' he said. 'I insist!'

I loved this guy.

But also: arrgh!

It was too late to argue, he was leading me towards the lift. He took me to his room, which was surprisingly small, with a single bed, and almost made me cry because it was so modest and childlike. He told me to make myself comfortable and said he'd wait down the hall.

I couldn't bring myself to sit on the bed, so I sat on the desk chair. I pulled out my breastpump and plugged it in. I attached the cup to my breast and fitted the fresh bottle to the other end of the pipe. I turned it on. *Week sqwawk, week sqwawk, week sqwawk.* It began to drain my breast. I watched the milk spurt out of my nipple, satisfyingly, in yellow-white jets.

My eyes wandered. I looked at all of my editor's things. The minutiae of his trip. His toiletry bag. His shirts hung up. A tote bag slung on the easy chair by the window. A view of the trees.

I think, *This is so normal it's lovely.*

I think, *This is the most abnormal thing.*

I think, *This is the most perfect symbolic representation of who I am now and the way all areas of my life and my past are joining up.*

I think, *This is fucking ridiculous.*

I think, *I'll have a glass of wine if my editor has one.*

I think, *I'll have a glass of wine anyway. Maybe two.*

I think, *What the hell am I going to talk to him about? I don't know about literary things any more and my brain is mincemeat.*

I think, *This is above and beyond contractual duty.*

I think, *Will he think less of me now?*

I think, *He never struck me as a man who uses Sure Cotton Fresh deodorant.*

But who am I now? I have no idea.

Wild Old Me

'He's a lunatic,' I say to Ian. 'He just wants to stay up all night. He's like some nocturnal maniac.'

I am talking about the baby. Ian looks at me. Because I am, first and foremost in life, a hedonist. I have chased feelings all over town. I am as good as one can be at hangovers. You'd think party girls would be good at late nights, at days without sleep. But no. No joyous bender or merciless come-down could have prepared me for this.

It will get easier, people keep saying to me. *When?* I reply silently. Now I realise they were talking in terms of years, not weeks. Because it doesn't get easier as the months pass. At four months, he's still up every few hours during the night. Sleep when the baby sleeps, they say. But when am I sup-posed to tidy, prepare for the next outing, wash myself, call my mum? I used to love sleep. 'She loves her feather,' my dad used to say. 'Sleeps on a washing line.'

But the tiredness is really taking its toll. I snap at Ian constantly. I hate him for getting out of all this scot-free, or so I see it. His body isn't injured. His brain isn't rinsed with hormones. But his OCD is creeping back. He has a touch of Tourette's – shouting random words as he walks around the flat. I hear him and I hate him for bringing more madness here. I have no space or compassion for him. Our love is breaking.

I want to be able to do everything. I want to be really good at everything. I want to do this right. But I am spreading myself so thinly. And then there is the admin. Dear god, the admin. I am the one who gets all the paperwork for appointments. I'm the one who keeps the diary. The one who counts the nappies and meals. It's my name on the maternity notes. My number with the health visitor. Ian texts me to check when appointments are. I am like the person running this show and delegating. I am management, he is staff.

Because it's not just the lack of sleep; it's the anxiety, the constantly looking after another person. The anxiety leads to a constant sense of doom. I am expecting something terrible to happen all the time. I am in a state of imminent catastrophe: Chicken Licken, waiting for the sky to fall. Keeping the baby alive is a major anxiety. I have one particularly vivid nightmare about him freezing to death. In the dream, I am with a friend staying in a remote cottage in the Lakes I used to go to, to write. We are having such a good time in the cottage that I leave the baby buggy outside the front door in the snow. The baby freezes. I wake up horrified, sweating, screaming. It's as bad as the dreams I had during pregnancy where I'd be at a party and hoover up a huge line of coke and someone would shout, WAIT, NO, YOU'RE PREGNANT! And I'd look down to see my huge stomach and – ohhhhh, Jesus.

I have daymares, too. Wicked waking fantasies. I think about letting go of the buggy at lights, and letting it roll into the oncoming traffic. I hate myself for these thoughts, obviously, but I cannot stop having them. In some ways I am torturing myself with my most dreaded thing, the worst event I can imagine, what my whole body is continually poised against – The Death of the Baby – but also, sometimes, at night when he will not sleep and he will not shush and my back aches and my head aches and I'm rocking rocking rocking rocking, it is my darkest, fleeting desire.

Amidst all this, Ian and I are still desperately trying to be normal: to be the couple we were; the people we were. We are also trying to find out who we are now. To join up the people we were before we became parents with the people we are as parents.

Then comes a rapid series of firsts.

Sex

Before this fateful night, it has been three months. Not a huge bout of chastity by modern standards, but a long period of abstinence for me and my partner. Will things be the same between us? Can passion coexist with knackeredness? Can passion coexist with having seen someone shit themselves on a hospital bed?

All of these questions have been rolling around, even if we haven't, so to speak. We did have sex during the pregnancy – possibly often as part of my rabid need to prove that I was the same person, that pregnancy wasn't going to change me. It was good to feel my body operating as *my* body – bump notwithstanding. Pregnancy sex also felt vaguely rebellious, and was better for that. It's the closest I've had to an orgy. Although Ian and I did seem to mysteriously turn into people with zero grasp of human anatomy. Will the penis bang the baby's head? Poke it in the eye? Should we wait until we think the baby is asleep? Should we be quiet? We googled, obvs. 'Your baby will have no idea what's going on,' said one of the websites, ominously.

After the birth, my vagina felt like mashed liver. Now I felt it on the toilet, horrified, intrigued, at this great change in me. I'd known I needed to give it time to recover, months and months, but I hadn't dared inspect it. I *had* checked that I could still have an orgasm. I masturbated, gingerly, three days after the birth because I was terrified I'd been stitched up incorrectly and I wouldn't be able to come ever again. My clitoris still worked, which was terrific news, but what was penetration going to be like? And why was I talking like an A-level biology textbook? Anyway, sex was off the menu those first few weeks. My tears and grazed labia meant I couldn't sit down, and peeing was like humping razorblades. The doctors came round to discuss contraception in the hospital a few hours after the birth. Haha! I like a health service with a sense of humour.

So, Tonight Is the Night. I've changed my knickers today and everything. But wait! I might have forgotten how to initiate sex. Certainly sober sex. Do I trust my body enough again to surrender to it, and let it feel its way? My body betrayed me during the birth. In her book *The Argonauts*, describing the birth of her son, Maggie Nelson writes: 'I like physical experiences that involve surrender. I didn't know, however, very much about experiences that demand surrender.' My body and I are in the process of becoming reacquainted. My partner and his penis are the same as they ever were.

In addition to this, I have a new penis in my life. I have grown one inside my female body. Penis envy is over. Now

I have a miniature penis to clean, several times a day. I have been near many penises in my life, but rarely in a cleansing context. It presents many challenges. For example, how does one clean a scrotum? It is dimply. A toothbrush would seem a good choice. A soft one, for sensitive teeth. The wipes don't always cut the mustard. (And newborn shit does look a *lot* like mustard.)

And there are other things that previously were sexual that have become functional and baby-related. My breasts are not an erogenous zone right now. I don't particularly want them touched. My nipples have only just recovered from the mastitis and thrush. Also, they leak. I often wake in a wet patch … of lactated milk. I have to wear breast pads in my bra. Sometimes the pads work their way up and poke out, coquettishly, in shops. That said, I'm pleased the baby is now feeding well. He isn't sleeping well, so it's good to have something. I like the complex, satisfying fact that my body is sustaining his body, even though he is outside of me now – and that dependency denies me my freedom. In the early weeks, nothing would quieten the baby other than feeding him, and it was a relief to know that something would always work. Although I did start accusing myself of 'throwing a boob at the problem'. I know that I am still often throwing a boob at the problem. My friend Rachel says this is my metaphor for life now. Truly at the nadir of my feminism, folks.

Also, I am not fully thinking about our birth control. Women more often than not manage the contraception in long-term relationships and after having a baby. I resent this and often argue with Ian about it. It's like the domesticity thing. It's like managing the kitchen but in your *own body*. Why should we do this? Yet we slip into it. Ian, a doctor, says the male pill didn't work because 'men can't be trusted to remember'. Fuck that! They have to be trusted. They have to share this load. We all have to share the load. And yet, I am the one taking the pill again. Considering a coil.

Back to the sex. So, we are naked. The baby is asleep. The lights are off. But wait! The old pregnancy worries come back to haunt us. Is it ethically dubious to have sex, with a baby less than a metre away? Will he know? Sometimes I think he's a sponge-in-progress; other times I think he is as smart as a smart dog. Would a smart dog understand sex? Would it care? I daren't google this. My search history is incriminating enough. And there's no way I'm taking this one on fucking Mumsnet.

'In the olden days, entire families lived and slept in one room,' Ian whispers, as though this is reassuring. I am a modern woman! Or I was, before all this.

The baby snores. We go for it.

It feels … different. Mainly because I have no pelvic-floor muscles. I'm trying to exercise them every day when I do other boring jobs such as make a cup of tea. I've put up Post-it notes around the flat to remind myself, that I then have to take down when people come round in case they think I'm some kind of pervert. But right now sex feels numb and poky, not clenchy and unctuous.

'Does it feel different?' I ask Ian. I hate myself for asking this; for succumbing to fears, but I want to know.

'No!' he says. It is the right answer. He is the right man.

It is quick sex – quick like meals are now, like everything is apart from the days alone with the baby, which are slow and long. It is sex like I had when I was drunk and not in love with people – clunky; emotionally distant – except everything is lit with stark, sober clarity. It doesn't connect us. It feels sort of tragic. I start to cry. Oh god, crying during sex – this is not good. This is a first.

'Are you okay?' Ian says.

'Yes, fine,' I say, 'probably just hormones.'

And who knows, maybe it is. Who knows anything any more.

It might also be that I feel far away from the man I used to love. Or that when we were trying to get pregnant, we tried not to try too hard. We tried to not let our sex be just about procreation; to preserve some part of us that was just for us.

In the middle of the night I get up to feed the baby and realise, en route to the feeding chair, that there might be a non-lactation-related wet patch on its way. I sit on a dirty AC/DC t-shirt. This gives me an indecent amount of satisfaction. Who says my rock 'n' roll days are over?

Cigarettes

Three months into new motherhood, I smoke my first cigarette in eleven months. It is delightful. I'm not going to start smoking again – not regularly, anyway. (I'm going to become one of those people who hawks round for cigs after a few drinks and never buys any of her own – it's payback time.) But this one is like a little stick of heaven. I blame *Before Sunrise*, which we watch after dinner. The ineffable cool of Julie Delpy and Ethan Hawke as they swan around Vienna having earnest conversations about life. Do you know how many people smoke in that movie? Loads. As I watched it, I felt the desire for a fag creep up my throat. I'm impressionable like that. It's a pretty good job it wasn't *The Wolf of Wall Street*.

I last until three-quarters of the way through the film, and then I turn and say to Ian, 'Mind if I have that cigarette?' Not because I need his permission, but – oh, maybe I do. It's a shared thing, the baby, after all – and everything that comes with him. I'm not sure where my body ends and the baby's begins yet. How much of me I own. What is polite, respectful, kind, motherly, allowed. I'm hoping Ian and I can navigate these strange new seas together. But then I know there's also a look in my eye that says, *I'm having that fucking cigarette, mate*.

'That' cigarette being the one in the box in the spare room on the bookshelf. It has been there since the day I found out I was pregnant. Before that, I was smoking five or six a day; more on a night out. I'm not judging women who smoke during pregnancy. I just didn't. I did fancy a cigarette during the last months and I resisted, but I've really been fancying one now the baby's here. I've been slowing my pace passing smokers in the street, pushing the buggy deliberately closer to them. Letting the silty entrails of their out-breaths hit the back of my throat. Swallowing luxuriously.

Watching *Before Sunrise*, I was jealous of their train journey, their freedom, their romance.

The thought of getting a train anywhere with the baby fills me with nerves. What if the baby cries incessantly? What if the baby shits everywhere? I always thought I'd be an intrepid mother, but somewhere since the birth I've become a real scaredy-cat, and it's like I've got to build up all my grit again. Maybe smoking is a good place to start. I've always felt good smoking. I love cigarettes like I love alcohol. They connect me to the tough teenager inside. The girl who felt like she could do anything, and often did. The cigarette in the box in the spare room is a menthol, like I smoked when I was a teenager, behind bowling alleys and on the top decks of buses. It was Consulate Menthols then. Now it's Marlboro Ice Blast. I pull it out of the box and smell it. It smells strong. Headache-inducing. I wonder how this will go down. Whether it is a bad idea.

There is a lighter on the windowsill that I have been using for scented candles. I grab it. I put on my coat, go out to the balcony, huddle myself on the bench and spark up. The first toke knocks my head back and my eyes close, like a doll's. I exhale, remembering how I was accused at school of 'not inhaling' – that terrible faux pas, worse than not having started your periods. The class bully once laughed at the way I held my cigarette – straight fingers rather than curled – 'like a fucking amateur'. I still hold my cigarettes like that. I am a fabulous fucking amateur. I happen to think it looks more elegant. The rest of the cigarette I smoke quickly and compulsively; like eating something luscious, there's pleasure in the sheer speed of consumption. I glance to the baby in the lounge, Ian next to him. It's not a big deal … or is it? It's so hard to know any more what is a big deal and what isn't.

The cigarette tastes sweeter, I am sure of it, after so many months of being told what to do. I think after pregnancy and childbirth you reach a point where you think, *I'm having something for me*. Like a pedicure. Or a cigarette. I've also been thinking a lot about how I can make the old me and new me align. Where they join. I chose this, but it's still overwhelming. The nebulous grey areas of my identity mix and blend, like a cloud of smoke around me.

Drugs

Around this time I get a group text from a drug dealer who evidently still has my number from a few years back, offering me 'Power for the weekend, if you need it, special offer, here with all the best w wine.' Lol. I've never needed power more. Some energy would be great too while you're at it, mate. Sadly, it's a euphemism.

I send my friend Sally a text to make her laugh: 'Having a baby is worse for your body than cocaine.'

I sort of mean it.

Other remnants of old me include an ecstasy tablet from my friend Maggie which she gave me as a Christmas present just before I found out I was pregnant. It is in the spare room, in a ring box, high on a shelf, nestled between books. More tantalising still, Maggie told me it was 'the best pill she had ever taken, as good as in the 90s', which is why she'd bought an extra one for me. It winks at me through the wall. I open the box periodically and look at it. I know that it is wildly inappropriate to keep this in the house 'as a mother', but I can't throw it away. Not that I'm going to do anything with it, of course. Jesus, I double-dropped my postnatal vitamin by accident and panicked I'd give him too much vitamin A through the breast milk.

Alcohol

I think a lot about my aunt's advice, dished out at Christmas when we were bemoaning what a bad sleeper he was, to just 'give him some brandy'.

I get drunk for the first time when my friend Maria comes to stay for the night.

I love booze. Booze is my drug of choice. My friend Rachel had actually deduced I was pregnant because I 'hadn't posted a picture of myself with a drink on Instagram for a week'. Booze is one of my greatest pleasures. Now my relationship with drinking has had to change for a while because someone needs me, and I don't need booze. I'm trying to judge the effect this might have upon my social life. Which parts of my identity will survive this new life phase, and which will have to be left behind? I don't want to be the same person for ever. Part of the definition of a living thing is to grow and move and change. So, the gauntlet is thrown. I'm waiting to see what comes out in the wash of motherhood.

At six weeks we had gone for dinner with our NCT friends Alex and Simon and then back to theirs for a nightcap. They are great people, warm company for a winter's night, and the nightcap turns into quite a few whiskies. It is wonderful. I don't even mind the slightly fuzzy head the next day. I feel, well, like me. Old me and new me can coexist. Hurrah!

However, the hangover with Maria is not so clever. I have had many boozy nights with Maria, we've been friends for almost twenty years, so there is an old Pavlovian excitement when we see each other. An expectation. Ian says he'll manage the babycare, and I'm not breastfeeding any more (we've put the baby on formula), so Maria and I polish off a few bottles of wine and start on the spirits. At a subconscious level, I am on some crazed mission to prove that I am still the same person, that I am not a mumsy loser.

I make Ian take a photo of us drinking out of champagne coupes and I post it on Instagram. Still fun! Still wild! Look!

Then Maria and I sit on the old wooden bench out on the balcony. We watch the buoy with the red light bobbing on the sea. I look further, as I always do, for lights of small fishing boats and passing ships on the horizon.

'How are you finding it?' she asks.

Maria has a son in his late teens. She had him when she herself was in her teens, and had to flee to a refuge because his father was abusive. I feel like I don't have problems. What the fuck do I have to complain about?

I look out at the sea. 'I'm fine,' I say, smiling. 'It's just … a bit restricting sometimes.'

'Motherhood is a natural disaster,' Maria slurs. 'It breaks your body.'

I look at her. She laughs lustily, like a pirate.

I look out to sea again. 'Beware all ye who enter here.'

'Too right.'

I don't have to get up in the night, but when Ian heads to work the next morning I realise my error. I hold it together while I play with the baby and put him down for his morning nap, and then I run to the toilet. A stray sock has found its way into my dressing gown and drops down the toilet into my wee as I stand there, waiting to puke. The sock suddenly appearing terrifies me, and it takes me a good few seconds to work out what it is and where it has come from. The shock makes my headache worse. I think, *This is so much worse than having a job because there's no one I can phone to say I can't do it*.

I make an attempt to tidy up, but realise I cannot take the bag of empty bottles out to the recycling bin because the neighbours know that I have just had a baby. Why did I advertise this fact? I chastise myself for my lack of foresight. For the same reason, I cannot open the kitchen blind until the dishwasher has finished and been reloaded because there is every kind of glass lined up on the work surface waiting to be washed: shot glasses, wine glasses, even a brandy glass that I was drinking whisky out of because I deemed 'thin glass makes it taste better'. Such a connoisseur. Only the postman, who has seen me in various states of disarray and emotion over the past ten months, doesn't bat an eye. For this, I love him.

I notice with alarm that the baby needs his nail trimming. There is no way I am up to this feat of neuro-surgical proportions. I wouldn't trust myself to cut my own nails today.

I puke in the shower, which makes sense from a cleaning-up point of view. There is a beautiful logic there. I feel as though I am rinsing away my shame. I do not know how the fuck I am going to change a nappy. I want someone to change my nappy. Just your regular Mother Earth.

Maria, who has puked six times in the toilet, emerges and accuses me of being 'a bad influence'. She doesn't make any of her meetings that day. This is like old times! Except …

One of the other mums I met on the NCT course WhatsApps the group to say she is going for a two-hour walk. Many say they will join her. I do not, for fear of reeking of alcohol and potentially having to puke behind a bin. My baby isn't getting as much fresh air as the other NCT babies today. I am despicable.

Maria goes back to bed. The bastard. I have the runs. I take the baby in his bouncer into the bathroom and put him at the far end while I horribly poo. The haemorrhoid makes an appearance. It feels like atonement.

I remember now that I smoked three cigarettes (*blargh*), and the memory of these is the worst thing. I reload the dishwasher and raise the blinds, leaving the Ecover dish-washer tablets out in full view on the windowsill to prove that I am a responsible person.

I feel so tired – like we partied until 4am. Apparently, we were in bed for 11pm.

I eat an entire pack of Choco Leibniz. They make me feel so much better that I want to write to the people who make Choco Leibniz and personally thank them. The Choco Leibniz hit my stomach and I feel sick again.

Because I cannot find any other socks, I put on the one that fell into the toilet. It dries by noon.

I think about how worried I was that having a baby would change me. Now I'm worried that it hasn't. Although in the mirror I do look a lot like a mumsy loser. Maybe I've achieved more than I know.

After this wretched morning, I wonder how much the party girl in me is fighting the new situation. I know I was frightened and feeling inadequate, and the teenager in me was rising up with fists. I recognise that motherhood is a major turning point I am not ready for. Is this what every woman, every parent, realises?

Rock 'n' roll

I try a baby group called Baby Sensory – which has a 'Rock 'n' roll Special'. Excellent! I sign up like an over-excited fresher, and somehow find myself singing 'hello to the sun and the corn', as balls roll around on a piece of taut neon voile. In all honesty I've had weirder Thursday mornings, but I've usually still been high. Bubble machines, balloons, light projections, cushions, maracas, confetti … Really, it would be the perfect environment for LSD. If the babies weren't there.

Baby Sensory is the first mother-and-baby class I've taken him to. It isn't always rock 'n' roll. That's just this week's theme. Next week it's superheroes. I lucked out. I go with one of the other NCT mothers, Lisa, who tells me on the way that during the past two classes she's taken her baby to, he screamed throughout one and slept throughout the other.

I don't know what my baby is going to do. He likes outings, he likes other people, but babies are so unpredictable. I feel unprepared.

I look down at my bags hooked onto the buggy, like that game Buckaroo. Nappy bag, check. Muslin, check. Extra muslin, check. (He's going through a pukey stage.) Change of clothes – *shit*. I knew I'd forget something. I look at the baby in his new M&S snowsuit. *Don't shit yourself*, I beg him with my mind. Or at least let's not have one of those whole-leg affairs. I don't know which of us is cleaner most days. At the cranial osteopath's I had baby sick in my hair from the previous day. I'd kept meaning to wash it out and just not got round to it. I realised I was a walking cliché: a new mother with sick in her hair. I can't even be revolting in an original way any more.

Baby Sensory is held in a church hall. There's a circle of mats and a few mums on their knees putting babies into position on the floor. I sniff the baby's trousers – the coast is clear so far, excellent – and put him down. He looks around at the other babies and then back to his hands. He has just discovered his hands. He spends much of the day waving them in front of his face, amazed, and staring at them like Kate Bush. Someone else's baby is already screaming the place down. The mother is walking the perimeter of the room, shushing him. Everyone is giving her supportive looks. There but for the grace of God, we all think. There but for the grace of fucking God.

The lady taking the class is called Aggie. 'Babies love music!' she says. 'Life without music is no life at all!' I like Aggie. She's wearing at least six different types of print. Aggie gives zero fucks. I myself am wearing sparkly trousers. Black with glitter in the fabric. The woman next to me admires them. I thank her. After a dabble with the bizarre burgeoning commodity that is maternity fashion, I'm back to expressing myself through my clothes, mainly because I'm usually too tired to actually speak.

We sing the 'Hello' song. I don't know this song, but it's easy enough to bluff. *Hello sun, hello moon, hello corn.* There are signs to accompany the words. My baby is mesmerised. I get emotional at the thought of him learning sign language. I'm ready to weep at most things at the moment. I keep crying at bank adverts. And I hate banks.

Then we get to the rock 'n' roll. We rock the babies from side to side, singing, '*There were ten in the bed and the little one said, roll over, roll over!*' I haven't heard this song for a while. The nostalgia is strong. I tell myself to absolutely not cry. Crying is not rock 'n' roll. Someone needs to tell the other woman's baby. He's still bawling his head off. She's breast-feeding, fruitlessly, while he claws at her hair. I ask her if she wants some formula. I have some in my bag. She doesn't, she says. She just wants him to fucking shut up. We're all with her. Solidarity against the babies, sometimes.

The maracas come out, along with a selection of home-made shakers. Coloured beans in plastic water bottles. We have two each. The babies are encouraged to hold them. My baby takes one in each hand and goes nuts. Several of the babies hate it and start crying. I can't say I blame them. It's a fucking cacophony.

For the final activity, we sit in a circle and hold taut between us a sheet of shiny blue fabric with holes in it, rolling bright pink footballs across and shouting 'HURRAY!' each time one goes down a hole, all to a soundtrack of 'Rock Around the Clock'. It's a song that reminds me of my dad. Then I really do start to cry.

Motherhood feels like a psychedelic adventure and I have always preferred fast drugs for the reason that I don't like fragmentation. I am not willing to go to pieces. I want things – people, drugs, songs, books – to say: *There you are. Stop. There.*

I do not know where I end or where I begin any more.

Note

For a second I think, *Has Ian killed him?*

For a second I think that's the worst thing.

For a second I think, *Oh, but the silence is beautiful.*

For a second I think, *Could we leave it two hours before we ring the emergency services, just to have a sleep?*

For a second I think I am a terrible person and a despicable mother.

A wail. Thank god. Oh god.

My heart sinks and leaps, sinks and leaps.

The Fizz

It's not often I develop a hatred for a children's TV character, but Jesus, I hated Upsy Daisy with a passion. I was so angry at her for having her bed on wheels to get in, alone, whenever she liked. To sleep alone in a field full of flowers. Imagine that bliss. Lucky bitch. *In the Night Garden* is torture for new mothers for this very reason. It is a taunt.

I really did think it was just tiredness. Extreme, unprecedented, soul-destroying tiredness. But as the new year turned into spring, what I was feeling became more than tiredness. It calcified into something deeper, darker, more lethal. While the world was getting lighter, my mind was going dark.

So hard to tell when the first real drops of the depression fell – those damp specks on the pavement; the subtle warnings of the oncoming deluge. When was that? What was that? Was it when I started feeling irritated by Ian almost every moment, and couldn't remember why we were even together? Or was it when I felt so out of control of the nipple pain I was in that I started doing silent screams while I was breastfeeding? Or was it when I started dreading going to bed rather than looking forward to it, because I was already dreading being constantly woken up and tortured, as well as being unable to get comfortable with my hips? Was it when there was no relief or respite anywhere at all? Nowhere safe to run. No possibility of running even if there was. Was it when I started feeling as though my career was over and would never recover? Or when I felt I had lost intimacy with all my old friends, and was a million miles away from my family? Or was it just when I felt – almost daily – as though I'd woken up in somebody else's life? When I started writing weird sentences and messages as though I wasn't in my mind and body any more?

All of those things, and more. It was a thousand tiny factors that built and built, grew and grew, accumulated into a mass. A cloud, coming to engulf me.

I remember one afternoon finding myself on my hands and knees on the floor of the kitchen, sobbing. I have no idea how I got there. I'd put the baby down for a nap and must have gone in there to make a hot drink, maybe – and the next thing I knew I was crying on the floor. It was like being black-out drunk and coming to in a taxi, or at a random party. Except I never got drunk like that. I always remembered everything. When people wanted to piece together the events of an evening, they'd call me. I remembered every segue, every plot point. My memory was rubbish in many ways – I often forgot films I'd seen or entire books I'd read – but I could remember how and when I got myself physically from A to B, always.

Not any more, it would seem.

Ian found me.

'What are you doing?' he said. 'What's the matter?'

I looked at the floor. It was disgusting, like the rest of the flat. I got up. I don't know why I didn't move towards him for a hug, or why he didn't move towards me. We were both bewildered by the whole situation, I think. I think I probably blamed it on the state of the kitchen, which was a surefire way to start an argument.

'Nothing is good enough, is it?' Ian said, like he always said.

It wasn't.

Nothing was good enough because everything was shit and dark and bleak and pointless.

'Please, please get some help,' Ian said.

'I don't need that kind of help!' I roared. 'I need someone to clean and tidy and look after ME.'

'That person does not exist,' Ian replied.

And so we went round and round.

There is a rather tired analogy that compares books with babies. The conception. The gestation. The labour. And so on. I can't help but think the analogy is in fact most pertinent in the context of keeping something alive. This thing will die if you do not tend to it. True of babies. True of books. For me, it was a question of absorption. Writing fiction requires a level of absorption of which I had known no like. Perhaps grief. Or lustful early love. I couldn't think about anything other than my son. I knew motherhood would involve sacrifices – of course it would – I had no idea how many sacrifices, or how huge they would be. My head was abuzz. I couldn't think and, for me, thinking is 90 per cent of writing. I felt as though I had made an exchange. I could not mentally sustain both a baby and a book. And so my book died.

I was terrified about money. I was not on paid maternity leave from a company. My money was running out. My office had become the baby's bedroom (classic). Not all women want careers. Many see motherhood as a career. Many choose motherhood and don't care about money. I respect all of those ways of living. But for me, what I sensed as a gross and growing unfairness spurred me to rageful thinking and frustration. Despair. Mania.

On some level I knew that I was fighting my own anni-hilation, and this was not a new fight. It was the fight I'd had every time I'd walked home through a dark park, every time I'd asked someone for something in a work situation, even though people with accents or backgrounds like mine didn't usually get places in the industries I wanted to work in. But this was my toughest opponent yet. Motherhood. Because wrapped up in it was my heart. I couldn't separate out the bits to bite and the bits to lick.

And underneath it all was some notion of my own responsibility in the matter.

'You are a massive over-achiever,' Katie said. 'Always have been, always will be.'

I am furious at this for a second. Because it's a criticism, and as a massive over-achiever I dislike negative criticism of all kinds. But when I think about it, she's right. I am a massive over-achiever. I put a lot of pressure on myself. To keep going. To seem in control. I felt as though I was being made to present as coping, but the idea of 'being made' to do anything is interesting. I see now that some of that was my own internal state, not just external pressures.

My nerves were a-jangle all the time. I had terrible thoughts. There was an energy in the air. A fizzing sleeplessness. A fiery restlessness inside. A malignant discontent. Electrical things seemed to break and bust all around me. The TV turned itself on and off randomly (or was I imagining it?). I was trained to jump – to fucking JUMP – whenever the baby made the slight-est noise. I don't know who trained me to do this. Or what.

One time I got stuck in the lift (the cursed, too-small lift in my block of flats) for five minutes with the baby when we were on our way out. It was terrifying. The lift just stopped. I was afraid, because being stuck in a lift is never nice, not to mention when your nerves are frayed, but also the idea of being trapped with the baby in an even smaller space than the flat was too much to bear. I punched the lift buttons uselessly. When nothing happened, I pressed the alarm button. The alarm didn't sound. Instead it went to a 'number not recognised' sound. I tried to phone Ian. I had no reception. The bile was high in my throat. After five minutes of staring at the baby, the baby staring at me trying to work out why I was so wide-eyed, why I was swearing at the building and all listed buildings in general because they can't have any improvements done to them like have the lifts enlarged and made actually efficient, or have doorways widened (we'd had to cut our sofa in half and then put it back together inside when we moved in), and are largely not fit for purpose and damp and draughty and— the lift shuddered to life and started moving again. I screamed. The baby stared at me. His eyes moved down my face, resting on my large chin-mole. I was getting paranoid about how much he was staring at my chin-mole. He had an obsession with my chin-mole.

When we got out of the lift, I pushed the buggy out to the street where – *splat* – a seagull promptly shat on my coat and the baby's changing bag. Truly my lucky day.

I joke about it now. But you know what, I didn't laugh at the time. I cried. Out of sight of the baby. And that should have been a big warning. In a way it was the cruellest part of the depression. It robbed me of my sense of humour.

A fizzle. A sizzle. I felt like I was always standing near a pylon.

The Cracks

And then it comes. The storm breaks.

First, I hit a wall.

One night the new neighbours start drilling holes in the wall at 8pm and the noise wakes the baby. Drilling at night is never welcome, but this sends me over the edge. I scoop up the screaming baby from his cot and – with him in my arms – I take a large antique hole-punch my father gave me, still on the shelf in here from when it used to be my office. (My spacious, peaceful office.) I bash the hole-punch repeatedly against the wall. I do it ten or twenty times. It makes a huge racket and the drilling stops. Meanwhile Ian has started running downstairs to tell them to stop. I keep bashing the hole-punch against the wall, over and over. The hole-punch makes large gouges in the paintwork and plaster. When Ian comes back up, he is horrified. I put the baby back in his cot and return, wordlessly, to the lounge. I feel a sense of being purged, and weirdly reassured. The rage, although frightening, is the only thing I have felt – physically, mentally, spiritually – in a long time. It tells me I am still alive. I can have an effect. I have power. The shards of adrenaline are like bolts of electricity, keeping the monster moving.

Second comes a storm from a teacup.

Ian reminds me he is going away for a few days. He has been invited to give a keynote talk at an academic conference in Berlin. It must have been a good day when I agreed to this. The conference is in a field he helped to found, so it feels important to him, and the baby is nearly a year old. We are sitting together in the lounge at night, drinking tea. When he tells me he is going away, I stare at him. The air between us is charged. I am processing this information. Or maybe not processing, because before I know it I hurl my half-full mug across the room towards him and it hits the wall. It smashes into brown and white fireworks. Ian leaps across the sofa, out of the way.

'What the fuck?!'

Did I mean to hit him? I don't know. Am I glad it smashed? Yes. Do I want to smash more things? Yes. Big style.

I have never been a crockery thrower. Never been one for violence, or confrontation even. But as I stare at the tea sliding down the wall in great dirty tears, at the thin shards of porcelain on the floor, I feel like I am on the edge, finally, of something truthful. I hate life, I hate Ian, and I hate the fact he can decide to go away for a few nights. Why is he not imprisoned, like me? I know I am also on some level terrified of being alone, of being left. I know that I cannot cope. The crying is getting more frequent. I am constantly on the edge of a psychotic fit. The friction between us is unbearable.

Then the anger leaves me, and I feel stupid, and needy, and pathetic. I am better than this! This is not me! I am a strong, independent woman. 'You can go!' I say. I don't want to be the bratty wife, the clichéd woman trying to keep him under the thumb.

As I'm writing this book, I can still see the sepia tentacles of the splash-stain from that night. If I walk into my son's room I can see the dents and gashes in the wall from the hole-punch. Three years on and we haven't redecorated. We have plans to move, but I also know I have left those reminders there to tell me something. Lest I forget.

The next thing that happens doesn't leave markers outside, but inside.

Ian goes away to Berlin for three nights. I am alone with the baby, with all the work, with my increasingly darkening brain. I am unslept, unwashed, unable to reach out to anyone.

The second day Ian is away, there is an afternoon where the baby won't stop crying. He cries and cries and cries and cries and cries. I think my head will burst. The baby is strapped in his buggy in the lounge because I am about to take him out for a walk to see if a change of scene will help, but he's crying and crying as I'm putting on my shoes and I want to fucking kill him, I do, I want to kill him, or anything to make the noise stop. What I have inside of me, this rage I feel, is not normal. It is a rage that transcends all motherly feelings. It is self-preservation and self-destruction in one. A deep, razing campfire in the pit of my heart.

Even now, years on, when I'm exhausted and he's misbehaving, a flash of this old rage sears through me, and I envisage spinning him round and round into walls, smashing his skull, silencing him. Ending him, and the stress. It's under control, and I am better now, but the darkest fantasies and desires, pure animal, pure ego, exist. I empathise with women who for whatever reason found such a thing got out of their control, for even a brief moment, and then lived to regret their actions for ever and ever and ever.

And.

And.

Oh god.

I don't want to write this, but I must. I must because I want to be honest, and say how bad it got, because I want women to not feel like freaks if they do or feel similar. It is a place where we need more support and should demand it. I also know now how much I love my son, to the point where it makes my heart explode, because I am well, and I know him, and now is not then.

But this is what happened.

The next night, Ian was still away and I was woken as usual every two hours or so by the baby. At one point I took him into bed with me because it just felt easier. When he woke me again a few hours later, he was sitting up in the middle of the bed, crying. I tried to give him his bottle. He didn't want it. He pushed it away. He continued to cry. God, I wanted to get away – anyhow, anywhere. Just away.

'*What?*' I shouted at the baby. 'What more can you possibly want from me?'

He sat there on the wide sheet, shaking, crying.

And then I reached out and I pushed him, hard, with my right hand. I was full of hate as I did it. I pushed him. It was enough to make him fall sideways on the bed.

I want you to know that it breaks my fucking heart to write this now. But I must write it, I think, for all the women who are at breaking point or who think they are monsters because they feel the violence rising. You are not monsters. You need more support. I must write it because it's the truth, and if we're going to move this conversation forwards we have to stick our necks out if we feel we can. So there it is. The worst moment of my life, the biggest weight in my heart, written in plain words on a page. I will resist the urge to delete delete delete.

The baby screamed like he was dying. He screamed like anyone would if their mother pushed them away in hatred.

I think something in me broke then, broke properly, because I picked him up and pulled him towards me and hugged him and said sorry and rocked him and cried myself. And maybe that's all he needed in the first place. A hug. Some reassurance in the night. But I was so cut off, so in need myself, so ill, I was blind to the most basic human things. When he had settled I laid him to sleep on Ian's side, and then I sat up alone in bed, wanting to kill myself. I started to feel angry again and, with nowhere else to direct it, sent Ian a barrage of awful texts.

I want to kill myself I hope you are having fun

I am going to go away next week just so you know

I want a divorce

That kind of thing.

He calls me. He is worried. I apologise, burnt out inside. I say the baby is sleeping, we are fine. I am just lonely. He believes me. He chastises me for sending him texts like that in the night. In a way, it's not his fault, because he doesn't know how bad I am. I am hiding so much, so much.

Now Ian tells me this was one of the worst times of his life, too. He was a mess and didn't know what to do, and was desperately ringing our friends for help and advice. We were so lost to each other, and both blinded by horrible anger. A wall of rage burned between us.

Years later, drunk and high on a hen-do, an old friend will tell me – shamefully, so shamefully – that when her daughter was nine months old she threw her on the bed in a rage. She says she couldn't take it any more. I say I understand. She cries. I try to talk to her about it again the next morning, sober, but she denies it. She says she blacked out.

A Playlist for the Worst Days

'Don't Walk Away' – Jade
'Tears Dry On Their Own' – Amy Winehouse
'Run' – Stephen Fretwell
'I Can't Go For That (No Can Do)' – Hall & Oates
'Storm Warning' – I Am Kloot
'That's the Way Love Goes' – Janet Jackson
'Don't Get Me Wrong' – The Pretenders
'Emotion' – Bee Gees
'Hand In My Pocket' – Alanis Morissette
'Goodbye to Love' – Carpenters
'Bloody Mother Fucking Asshole' – Martha Wainwright
'Here's Where the Story Ends' – The Sundays
'Crazy To Love You' – Leonard Cohen
'Did I Ever Love You' – Leonard Cohen
'Going Home' – Leonard Cohen
'Master Pretender' – First Aid Kit
'Diamonds & Rust' – Joan Baez
'Safe Travels (Don't Die)' – Lisa Hannigan
'Rise Up With Fists!!' – Jenny Lewis and the Watson Twins
'Chicago' – Sufjan Stevens

'Pegasi' – Jesca Hoop
'Hearts and Bones' – Paul Simon
'See You Sometime' – Joni Mitchell
'Hey Mama Wolf' – Devendra Banhart
'She Belongs to Me' – Bob Dylan
'Roxbury' – DJ Yoda feat. Edo. G and Nubya Garcia
'More Than This' – Roxy Music
'Zoom' – Fat Larry's Band
'We Let The Stars Go' – Prefab Sprout
'It's My Life' – No Doubt
'Wichita Lineman' – Glen Campbell
'Is That All There Is?' – Peggy Lee
'Somewhere In My Heart' – Aztec Camera

Blue On Blue

I know things, myself, are not right now. But I still can't talk about it. I am dragging myself around in a dead sort of dream. A dying sun in a cold universe. Every time I turn, I spit out the odd fireball. But otherwise I am cooling, sad and lost. I limp around the streets, alternating between apathy and fury. People rave about Brighton's architecture. The buttercream Regency squares. The building we live in, Embassy Court, was built in the 1930s. It's all grey and white and pale yellows. Ian thinks it is serene, like a ship. He specifically wanted to live in it. To me it is ugly. It is bone, plasma, brain tissue, prison. A hard, brutal cell.

I am giving up on even seeming okay. I don't phone anyone and I don't take phonecalls. I've never been a fan of phonecalls but now I actively avoid them. I don't even know who to be any more when I'm talking to anyone anyway. My poverty of spirit is so great that I can't even find the right version of myself to hate vengefully and fruitfully. It is the feeling of surrender. I have given up. Apart from the odd spike of rage, I am flatlining.

Ian keeps saying I am like a black cloud, and I know I am. I feel like I barely know him. The whole relationship feels like a mistake and I am googling 'divorce' with a fruity mix of keywords daily, terrified in the knowledge that I have no financial independence to survive on my own – just a swinging caravan of debt. That is when Ian tells me more than once that I am 'almost psychotic' and begs me to get help. I refuse to listen to him, my rage compounded by the fact that, as a man, he has no idea what I am going through. I hate him for not having his body ripped apart during childbirth. I am angry he isn't ravaged by hormones. I envy what I see as his male privilege; his freedom from the situation. But he is terrified. I can't see it, but he is terrified. He doesn't know what to do. And terror is not a feeling often found in love.

Ian is unwell, too. His carefully managed OCD, a feature of his life since childhood, is taking control of him again. When he was a child it manifested as having to repeat phrases in bed at night in order to keep his family safe. When we were pregnant it started to creep back because he was anxious about caring for our new little family. It revolves around ideas of luck, magic, religion and the occult. I have some vague sense of Ian's distress, but it just annoys and inconveniences me. I also think he's just trying to get a grievance in when really he has nothing to complain about. Now his OCD manifests in repeated phrases, said out loud, at all times of day. He says some phrases fifty or sixty times a day. He will shout, involuntarily, expletives which make me jump. I hate it, because it shows his weakness too, and I know that one of us at least needs to be strong to hold the fort. I also have zero compassion in my heart right now, and maybe I hate myself because I am subconsciously aware that this is inhumane.

In one of his meanest moments, Ian accuses me of having a baby just to have something new to write about.

I am massively offended by this. I go and write about how massively offended I am by this.

Still, I know that this is the mean voice in his head, just as I have one in mine. The voice that gives him hell. It is trying to give me hell too. They go inwards and outwards, those kinds of voices. They do not discriminate. They spray hate.

We are both lost in our private madnesses; both flatlining, devolved and dying. How can we have this brand-new life amongst us and feel so … dead?

And then one Sunday afternoon, we go for a walk in the countryside with some friends. I don't want to go, don't want to see anyone – in fact I've cancelled on this couple twice before in the past few months – but Ian insists.

'You like them,' he says. 'And there will be bluebells.'

There are bluebells. Thousands of them. Blue on blue. Isn't it great when real life provides the right backdrop? And he's right about the friends, too, Alex and Stef. They are undemanding. They claim nothing of us. They are loving, giving people – they gave us the crib we have for the baby, in fact, and they wouldn't take any money for it and even bought a new mattress for when they gave it to us. Good sorts.

We meet them up on the South Downs, in a farmer's wood that has been opened especially for bluebell season.

I walk with Stef. I hang back a little. I am slow at walking these days, my hips still hurt, and I have the remnants of a relaxin-induced waddle. Stef waits for me and matches my pace. Stef has a bodyful of arty tattoos to die for, works for a charity that protects women from domestic violence, and reads more than anyone else I know. Ian pushes the buggy ahead with Stef's husband and their two young boys, who coo over the baby and jump around.

Stef asks me how I'm doing and I give her the party line. I'm fine. And then, out of nowhere (although is anything ever really out of nowhere?), she tells me the story about how she became mentally ill after the birth of her second son, three years ago. She tells me how she felt bleak and hopeless and like nothing would ever be good again and like she had nothing to look forward to, and at the same time horribly guilty because she was supposed to be being a mum. A glad, grateful mum at that. This shakes me to the core. It feels like a secret confession from one of the strongest, coolest women I know. I sense her shame, and I hate her shame.

'I didn't know what was wrong with me,' Stef says. 'And I didn't know how to get better.'

I listen to Stef and I nod my head, and I look at the bright swathes of bluebells and I move my feet along the thin white gravel path. I am functioning. I am a human, functioning.

'I had postnatal depression,' Stef says. 'It's really common.'

I think, *How sad, how sad for you, but not me – no, this is not me.*

I want to say, *Did you hurt him, did you ever try and hurt him, did you hate your husband, did you want a divorce?* Instead, I make all the right conversational moves. I adhere to the dumb etiquette of my carefully practised deceit. I ask her how she got over it. She tells me she found an incredible therapist, a specialist in family issues, who understood where she was coming from.

'Who was she?' I say.

I am intrigued, even though I am dubious about therapists. I am a writer (or I used to be), and I had this arrogant notion that I already knew how to process my thoughts and feelings through words. What could therapy offer? I already verbalised my feelings and reaped the benefits of that. I think I was also sceptical about the notion of 'closure'. I wasn't sure I believed in it. I think I have always thought that psychological progress is more a case of assimilation: you assimilate a bad experience, and you carry on. There are no neat endings. It's not like a book. An ex of mine also had his therapist come on to him, which made me doubt the profession somewhat. But I am not really writing any more. I am not doing anything.

Stef pulls a little blue business card out of her pocket. It has the therapist's name, number and email address on one side, and an impressionistic picture of the sea on the other side.

When we get home, for the first time a little voice somewhere inside me says, *Maybe? Maybe you? Maybe this?*

But no, not depression. I have never been depressed! I am not a depressive type. I attract depressive types, but I am not one.

I am still not ready to interrogate it, or maybe not capable of interrogating it.

Until the Mini convention. That fateful May day when I get lost and found, by Ian and my feelings. And I cry and cry over a burger I don't want and I say *Okay, okay, maybe I'll try and get a diagnosis.*

After the Mini convention, I find the business card Stef gave me, and I email the therapist, Kim. I say 'Hi, I'm not entirely sure I'm depressed, but you came highly recommended, so could I come in for a chat?'

Casual as you like.

Kim replies the same night. She says sure, and she tells me her terms and her rates. We make a date for later that week.

The Eye

The baby and I sit next to each other on the sofa one day. We regard each other. Suddenly, he points his index finger towards my face. I watch his tiny fingertip as it advances, unsure whether to stay there and risk an eye-poke. He's poked me in the eye before. He loves eyes, this kid.

His finger reaches my face and moves downwards towards my chin. I brace myself. A mouth-poke, maybe?

And then he presses my chin-mole, the thing he has been obsessing over for months. SQUIDGE.

I laugh. I am outraged, delighted, outraged. He doesn't laugh. His concentration intensifies. He keeps pressing it. Squidge squidge squidge.

I know that this is barely an act of love. He is merely fascinated by an imperfection; that for him this is curiosity, interest in my defect. I go with it, enjoying the contact, the connection, the feeling. He continues to press the mole over and over. Squidge squidge squidge squidge.

There you are. Stop. There.

The Sea

Kim lives along the seafront, towards the lagoon. I enjoy the walk there, alone, listening to music and just letting the sun hit my face and making me feel something simple, warm and physical. I am nervous about what I'm going to say, nervous about whether she'll be any good, nervous about going down on some kind of record. I know I'm late to therapy. It's sort of retro to be into therapy now, like vinyl. In fact, I'm so late to the therapy party there's an empty treatment room with a few trailing streamers, a dimp-filled punchbowl, and Freud and Jung passed out on the floor next to a half-deflated inflatable cock and a Gabrielle album.

Kim's house is like the houses I used to draw at school. Bay windows, a porch, a car in the drive big enough for a dog in the back and tents for camping trips. I knock on the front door first, incorrectly, not spotting her practice room round the back. A dog barks behind the door. She answers after a few minutes and tells me to head around the back. I crunch round on the gravel, already on the back foot.

She opens the door to a small extension just down the short drive. I step up two steps. She is wearing simple, loose clothes – a pale blue shirt and navy slacks. She has glasses and a heart-shaped face. There is a chair for her on one side of the room and a small sofa with hairy cushions on the other. She motions to the sofa for me to sit down. I sign some forms, a contract, a promise, and then we begin.

The room is cool and quiet. I look around, trying to find details of her life to draw on, to align myself with, so that she might like me more. I am like the detective in *The Usual Suspects* when Keyser Söze has left the room. I am piecing a life together from the fragments. But instead of solving a crime, I am pouring everything into an insatiable hole of social need. I am good at this creative, self-destructive shit. I stop myself. I am not here to be liked. I am not here to fit in. Besides, knowing me, this is some kind of elaborate procrastination to stop me tending to the matter in hand.

Kim has a look that makes me feel seen, right the way through. In the nicest possible way.

She is practised in the art of silence. I gabble into the dead air. I splurge it all out to Kim that first session.

'You talk very fast,' she says.

'Do I?' I say. I had no idea.

Initially, I am defensive. I tell her I don't believe in closure and I don't want to get 'better'. 'Getting better' is a patriarchal narrative and a marketing invention. Messy women are as valid as any. Women are not problems to be solved.

Kim looks at me.

'Of course I do want to get better, for me,' I say. 'But not to be more pleasing and palatable, you understand?'

She stares. Tough crowd.

I try jokes instead. 'I feel like I'm in an abusive relationship,' I say. 'He tortures me every night with sleep deprivation. He waterboards me with his sippy cup. He will not let me eat or drink or – lately – leave the room. I am captive to his every whim. I am at the mercy of a despot. A smiling assassin. He comes at me with the most beatific grin – and then socks me in the neck and goes for a double eye-gouge. How is this acceptable? Is there a number I can call? Like Childline, but for parents? Parentline. Hello, I'm being abused by my nine-month-old …'

There is a quiver of a smile at her lips, but no more.

I am going to have to give this woman more, dammit.

I am not a person who readily admits she needs help. I am proud. I like to be seen as someone very capable. But this is not about how Kim sees me. She is facilitating, refereeing, umpiring me with myself on a neutral playing field. The therapist is there but also not there. This is an empty space, a void, or the closest you could get to a void, to pour thoughts into and watch them hang together and then dissolve.

So I describe what I've been feeling. I tell her about the constant frustration, the crying on the kitchen floor, the irritability, the negative outlook that makes me feel doomed – and the crushing guilt that I should just be feeling very lucky for having a healthy baby, and any baby at all.

'I just feel like my head is too full, of worry and things that need doing for him. I'm expected to do everything and be okay and feel joyous and complete. But we are far away from both our families, so we don't have any support. I haven't had any proper sleep or rest for so long. And I have work deadlines because I didn't want to say no, as the projects were my passion, and it has taken me twenty years to reach a point where I'm paid to be a full-time writer so it feels hard-won. My partner is a huge support but he also doesn't get it, and he's been away, and—'

Kim nods and gives me a grim but kind smile.

'How bad has it got?' she asks.

I am not ready for this question. I look down. Here I am, at an impasse. I cannot tell her about the rage, the violence. What if she has to tell child protection? That old bedrock of fear: *They will take your baby away.*

'I have … been upset around him,' I say. I weep effortlessly as I'm talking. I shake my head. I can't say more.

She nods again and looks sad for me.

I feel defeated, but I also feel like it's a start. I have started talking. I am scratching the top off, and I will go deeper. I will call it by its name, like you do with any illness, disease, demon, storm. I haven't said the words 'postnatal depression' yet but they are swirling in my head.

'I don't know whether it's even appropriate to ask you for a diagnosis,' I say. 'But my partner thinks that might be helpful—'

Kim just nods.

'Do you think I have …?' My voice trails off.

I don't need to say it. She swoops in to save me. Kim tells me that, in her opinion, what we call 'postnatal depression' is an umbrella term for a variety of mental illnesses that she believes are 'a reasonable response to the demands of motherhood in the Western world'.

Imagine that. Everything I have been feeling – the anger, the panic, the outrage – is REASONABLE.

This is a revelation. It is the start of my recovery.

Something clicked into place that day, with those words. Enough for me to feel accepted, understood, and not alone. It was something like safety. Safety was something I hadn't felt in a long time. It was a good start.

As I start to grow stronger, Kim starts to challenge me, which I like. Why am I taking on so much more of the mental load than my partner? How have we allowed this to happen? My partner and I are both feminists. We both thought I could do everything. I realise that the idea of 'having it all' is a golden myth of modern Western motherhood. You can't have it all. No human can.

Now, I know that therapy isn't about endings. It's more about embracing the messy middle we're all living in (the bit writers hate writing) and saying to yourself, *This is how it is today*. It wasn't defeat. It was a positive step towards recovery. I suppose I felt traumatised, and because of that I felt like I was losing control of my life, and I didn't know how to take back that control because my usual way would be to write, but I was too tired, and too frightened that my writing meant nothing now, and too scared that everything I wrote felt public somehow, and too damn confused to even begin with a sentence that might be the start of any form I've ever known, even a diary entry. I had no way to let the words just pour out, which was what I needed to do. What we all need to do.

One day, walking back from therapy, I lie on my back on the beach and close my eyes. I listen to the amniotic swoosh of the waves on the shore. I look up at the clouds. I feel the wind. All of these things give me something. I savour it today. I am no longer a person who expects to intellectualise every experience in order to assess its value. I know there are things that will heal me and help me that I cannot quantify. Looking at a tree. Listening to the sea. Deep down, I have always known these things. I am the daughter of a devout naturalist. I fell out of more trees than I had hot dinners as a child. I was always scaling a rock or saving a bee. Nature turned against me after I became a mother. It crushed me. Now, nature helps bring me back.

I am accepting the 'natural disaster' of it, as Maria put it. Motherhood is seismic. It cracks open your life, your relationship, your identity, your body. It features the loss, grief and hardship of any big life change. I see now that I have to separate my relationship with motherhood from my relationship with my son, which sounds like a paradox, but is actually the only way I can process it.

At my next session, Kim asks me why I am trying to combine all areas of my life. I can keep the writing part of me separate from the mother part of me. It doesn't all have to slot together. She tells me to get an office, pronto.

I tell Kim how I thought the baby would fit around my world.

'You fit around each other's worlds,' Kim says.

I realise that the baby and I are learning how to be together. I had a stupid misconception that I had to be perfect for him, and that he would arrive perfect. I was so wrong. We are both just humans, learning how to be humans in a new relationship. Perfection does not apply.

But not having thought it through is common, and understandable. How can you prepare for something so seismic and unimaginable? We live in a culture that tells women they can do it all, but doesn't pay them as much as men. A culture that wants women to abandon their work and mother full-time, especially self-employed women like me. It's not as though the system supports us.

I know I was lucky to be able to afford therapy. It is available on the NHS but there are waiting lists and often group options are all that there is a budget for. But I'd say try it – and get a recommendation. I still have it regularly. Therapy was artless. It was a space I could fill with words that would never go further. Motherhood is sold as such a celebration – such a pure unadulterated joyous thing. But it is a mix of emotions for all of the mothers I know. It is okay to mourn your former life. It is okay to simultaneously embody grief and gratitude. It doesn't have to be all positive. I love my son dearly. But I have lost things, too, in the process of becoming a mother.

Therapy also revealed to me that I hadn't negotiated anything with myself or my partner before the baby arrived, in terms of time, space, headspace, privacy, weekly structure.

I had been very naive. My focus was on being the perfect mother, and while I was focusing on that, I was ignoring my storeroom of feelings.

I was my own worst and harshest critic. But here was something I had to do too. Give myself a goddamn break. Maybe tell the critic in me to hush up awhile and let the friend in me step forward, the part of me that would just be loving and kind and patient. The part of me that was capable of mothering me. She was the one I could trust with all this. I could just sit there and pour it all out on the rug in front of her and she would just look at it and hug me and say, *So what? You're still my hero*. We all have that part of us. We can all mother ourselves that way.

Over the next few months, Kim helps me piece together a sense of what I'm feeling. Why I'm so angry. Why I hate everyone and everything. Why my previous positivity has shrunk to a black hole of despair and fury. Why I feel, for the first time in my life, like it would sometimes be easier to just be dead. (At least then I could sleep.)

Every time I feel myself getting frustrated, Kim's words ring in my head: 'A reasonable response'. I am fucked, but it hasn't happened because I am weak or stupid or monstrous or mad. It is because I could never have coped with the amount life has flung at me. What I am feeling is mad, but it is reasonable. I have a mental illness, but it is a logical place to end up, somehow, given the circumstances. Someone understands how I have got there.

Then our neighbour Rosemary, a maternity nurse and nanny who lives in the flat above, offers to help out for mates' rates. The first time she takes him, I go and stand in the entrance of the supermarket, behind a trolley, alone. Not even moving. Just revelling in being ... alone, without responsibilities.

Over the next few months, I keep the therapy every week, I get time on my own as Rosemary takes the baby the odd day, and the sleep deprivation gets incrementally better. These are baby steps back towards mental wellness, but they are steps. I feel like I am coming back.

The Silver

The therapy is helping and I am getting more sleep, but I'm not quite there. I'm still angry and crying more than feels right, so I go and see my GP. I am reluctant to go on medication. I worry it might curtail my highs as well as my lows, leaving me stranded on a dull, flat middle ground of emotion. But I feel like I might need a chemical jump-start, and my GP agrees. The pills, Citalopram, work almost instantly and I start to feel more positive and capable. At first I hide the pills in my toiletry bag, stuffed in my glasses case. But as I get stronger, I leave the packet in plain sight. I need them like I need my glasses, to fix a bit of myself that doesn't work as well otherwise. There should be no shame in that.

I start working on the foundations of myself – that's how it feels, rebuilding myself from the ground up. I appreciate the benefits of exercise properly for the first time in my life. I start running. I have to redefine my relationship with alcohol. Alcohol affects your sleep, and sleep was the thing I needed to prioritise to properly reset my health.

Perinatal psychiatrist Dr Rebecca Moore says: 'There's no doubt postnatal depression is linked to sleep deprivation as sleep deprivation affects every single one of us. And then it becomes a vicious circle. You start off being sleep deprived, then you get depressed, then you really can't sleep and then you've got this horrible loop of not sleeping. With all my antenatal women I have big discussions about, How are you going to manage your sleep? What is that going to look like for you? What if your mental health is deteriorating to the point where you need to mix-feed so that your partner can use a bottle – have you thought about that? Sometimes you might have to stop breastfeeding if it's impacting on your mental health too much. Not everybody can sleep in the day and not everybody can sleep when their baby sleeps. So I think it would be better if we had a lot more of these honest conversations around sleep.'

It's a skill, learning how to sleep in the day, learning how to grab moments of relaxation. I feel like I am looking after the machine of myself. Not taking my body for granted any more.

I have physio for my hips, which doesn't work, so I have an MRI scan, which reveals a pre-existing severe scoliosis (a twist in my spine) and a deteriorated disc. The consultant says to keep my spine mobile and exercise as much as possible. To build up my strength. Building up my strength is very much the order of the day.

I remember the day I start loving my life again. I've been on the anti-depressants a month or so. The day isn't eventful otherwise – I am just sitting with my son on a bench near the beach while he eats an ice cream, and it is honestly as though the sun comes out in my head. I sigh and look up because it feels like some sort of deliverance, even though I'm not religious. Suddenly, everything feels possible rather than impossible. Everything feels hopeful rather than doomed. I want to smile at people who walk past rather than punch them. I know I can handle what is still hard, but not beyond my capabilities. I kiss my son's head and whisper: 'God, I love you. I'm glad we made it.'

For my son's first birthday party I hire a church hall, order ten bottles of prosecco, do a buffet and invite everyone I know in Brighton. As we're setting up I realise I am throwing a party for myself, too. To celebrate my own survival, as much as his. I can't believe a whole year has passed. I know they'll go faster and faster, too. As Auden said: 'The years shall run like rabbits.' Alex has her own take on it. She says: 'The nights are long but the years are short.'

I am still exhausted most of the time, but I feel as though it's acceptable to admit this now. To say I need help and support. To let people in, rather than keep them out. What has happened is not my fault. It is not me. It was something that happened to me, but I am getting out of it, slowly but surely.

In December, Ian takes me to see the murmurations of starlings that swirl over the sea every night before they roost under the old pier. They are magical. They scatter and gather like clouds. A living storm. Ian and I hold hands as we watch them. Dusk falls, and the baby nods off in his buggy. I used to think love was like the sun, constant and unfaltering: Shakespeare's 'ever-fixed mark, / That looks on tempests, and is never shaken'. Something that would stay steady my whole life. Now I know that love is not passive; it is active. It's that line in the Massive Attack song that talks about love being a doing word. Love is intelligent. It is knowledge and work. I only see the full arc of my love for Ian now. Rocking the baby when he wouldn't stop screaming the first night because he was starving and we didn't know what was wrong.

Ian's stamina, strength, endurance. The man, like me, climbs mountains. It isn't all smart conversation, or nervy thrills, or even getting each other's jokes all the time, it is someone who'll meet me in the middle, and show up, and keep showing up. Someone whose ego isn't based solely on external adoration. Those men are hard to find. Love is a growing, living, moving, breathing thing – and you have to water it, and give it space, and sometimes put it in a completely different area of the garden to make it happy.

There's a line in the film *Meet Joe Black* where Death, aka a hokey, peanut-butter-scoffing Brad Pitt, asks another character, Quince, how he knows his wife loves him. Quince replies: 'Because she knows the worst thing about me and it's okay.' It's a sentiment that moved me the first time I saw what is otherwise a pretty terrible film – and it's a line I think of often in recent years, when I feel like I have some sense of what that worst thing might be.

I hadn't really known the extent of my own depths until I experienced PND. I used to think my depths were a playful gothic wonderland decorated by Tim Burton that I could prance around in. But my true depths were confusing and terrifying – like falling into water when you don't know which way is up. I know that no one has ever seen me the way Ian saw me during that time, screaming and crying and throwing things around. Calling him every name under the sun. Our relationship was an awful place to be. But then, I was an awful place to be. I felt uninhabitable. For the first time in my life, I didn't love anything. The loss of love was the loss of self. How can you love anything when you don't know who you are any more?

When you break in front of someone there is a new

intimacy on the other side. During the PND, the main thing Ian and I were unable to give each other was friendship. Friendship now is what we work on the most as we continue to recover. The daily micro-tendernesses and kindnesses that take the weight off another person. Long-term love is active. It is intelligent. It is work. The PND felt like something that happened to me, but my love with Ian is not. It is not passive. It is not lust, or a fairytale romance. It is something I have chosen to do, and it is something I choose, over and over – every time I take a breath and pause before I launch into an old argument cycle, or I cook him his favourite meal when he's had a bad day, or get up with our toddler and let him have a lie-in when I know he's exhausted. He still gets up in the night when my hips are sore. There is power in that, and pleasure, and strength, and expansion. Part of my ongoing disentanglement from the illness is to look at what I was choosing and what I wasn't; what I could control and what I couldn't. I don't recognise the woman I was back then. I see pictures of her and I don't remember them being taken. Ian helped me return to myself.

There's a line in one of my favourite poems, by Anne Sexton, about how 'the worst of anyone can be, finally, an accident of hope'. Ian and I decided to become parents because we thought we'd enjoy it, and be good at it, and it's harder than we ever imagined, but also a greater love than we ever could have imagined, too. We recreated each other, and our love, in a return journey from Hell. And now when I look back, and down, I see fibres I can count and name, binding us together and holding us up. It isn't a pretty haze; it's a tough net of commitment and investment. Something I can really rely on.

I can remember now, quite clearly, the image of Ian putting the baby down that first night we came home from the hospital and I was in a daze. 'There we are,' he said as he laid him in the co-sleeper. He said it so gently. He still says that now, and I have started saying it too. 'There we are.' It is the most soothing sound in the world. It is the sound of my home.

I notice more and more about my son. I start loving the way he laughs in his sleep. A rich, lusty gurgle, just as he's dropping off. How have I missed this? It is incredible.

I start looking for the positives rather than the negatives. They are always there. My old positivity starts lighting my head up again. When I find a swim class that is starting just as we arrive, instead of feeling unlucky, I feel lucky. Previously, even if I'd made the class, I would have felt stressed or harassed because I dropped a towel, or forgot my bra, or because he was crying. It was all too much. The depressed mind clings to the notion of curses. Of doom. Of terrible fate. It's bullshit. But it is powerful bullshit when you are in its grip.

Other times, when card machines don't work in cafés and I can't get lunch, for example, I share his sandwich and snacks. That's fun. I focus on the good stuff, like how he plays in the café play area. I notice how he is a lovely, gentle boy with other children. He makes me proud. He shares. He greets. He gives all the teddies a bit of his biscuit.

As I chill out, he chills out.

And then, at last, he starts sleeping through. After three nights in a row of him sleeping from 7pm to 6am we want to cry with relief. If we go to bed at ten, we can get eight hours. Sweet fucking hallelujah. I still wake a lot in the night.

Sometimes he cries once and then settles himself. Sometimes it is as though our energies wake each other – and they still do almost four years on. We are still deeply connected.

One particularly hard day I was wearing something I'd worn three times already that week and I just needed to get out because we both needed the fresh air. The baby was making the series of little high-pitched sounds he often makes in his buggy when we're out for a walk. A series of *oooohs* and *aaaahs* and *eeeehs* and *boooos* that I had completely normalised.

An old man was walking along the seafront. (I know this sounds like a parable, but I swear it happened.) The man stopped as he walked past. I stopped too.

'Is he singing?' the man said.

I registered what the man was saying. He was talking about the baby.

'Yes,' I replied, because it struck me at that moment that it was exactly what the baby was doing.

The old man looked delighted. He reached into his pocket and pulled out a coin. 'I like to do this with babies,' he said. 'I give them a little silver coin, for luck for the family. Would that be okay?'

'Er … yeah, I suppose so,' I said.

He rubbed the coin against the baby's hand and I wondered for a moment whether this was appropriate, and then he curled the baby's hand around the coin and waved goodbye to us both.

I waved, and then as soon as he was a suitable distance away, I pulled the coin out of the baby's hand. Choking hazard, definitely.

I text Ian. 'The strangest thing just happened … He sings x'.

Ian replies: 'I know x'.

We shared a moment of real joy about that.

I held the coin in my hand all the way to the shop, then mindlessly put it in my purse with all the other coins. As I came to pay at the till, I realised.

'Shit!' I said, seeing there were three new ten-pence pieces in there, all identical. Which one was the lucky one? There was nothing else to do but keep them all.

When I got home I put them on a shelf of the typesetting tray of precious things we've hung in the hallway of the flat. A stack of silver, representing an old man's good wishes, and my addled mind. When Ian got home, he asked where the lucky coin was. 'It's there,' I said, 'in with all the others, somewhere.'

'Perfect,' Ian said. Because it was.

The Wash

But it's not all magical old men and loving texts. The road to recovery is uneven. There are dips and setbacks.

There is one particularly dreadful night where I drink – a *lot* – on my anti-depressants and end up AWOL in Soho for two hours. Friday 12 January. It is etched on my mind. I had coffee with a friend who was about to go into rehab and then, the other extreme, a boozy lunch with a friend at Quo Vadis (my new thing, the acetone and other breakdown products of alcohol would be mostly gone by the time I went to bed). The lunch turned into an animal session, where I pissed off two drug dealers and ended up at another friend's house, speaking in tongues.

The next day I woke up – I got home, thank god – with a sprained, swollen ankle and bruises all over my feet. I had many messages from concerned friends, and a string of WhatsApp messages from an extremely fucked-off drug dealer. The scariest thing about it was the blackout patches. I could not remember parts of the evening. Getting the sprained ankle. Getting to the friend's house. Getting home. This was something I had *never* had before. I usually remembered everything. My friend Alison told me I'd been slurring when she spoke to me at 4.30pm. I could not remember phoning her.

Ian was very understanding and took the baby for a bike ride so I could groan and reflect. He told me I was a wally for drinking on anti-depressants, but I really didn't know – I hadn't read the small print. I felt stupid and ashamed, and this time rightly so.

I liked being bold and wild. But we need to find new ways to be bold and wild, as well as the old ways we know. What happened that night wasn't fun. It was just frightening.

A big turning point is a writing retreat at a cottage in the Lakes with my friend Jesca. We go for five nights. It is the longest I've been away from my son so far. I turn up spotty, tired and already feeling guilty. Desperate to write but also desperate to jump on the next train home. Jesca takes one look at me and runs me a bath. She drops lavender and vetiver oils into it. It is the beginning of her self-care offensive. She gives me a pack of beeswax candles to write by.

She makes nourishing meals – things you couldn't whiz up for a baby afterwards. Divinely grown-up food: poached eggs on wilted greens with pumpkin oil and seeds. Roasted yams with quinoa, ancho chillies and sour cream. Chicken and cashews with black pepper. Rare roast beef and mustard. She gives me a strange calcium-magnesium drink every night before bed to relax me. It tastes like chalk but I sleep like a baby. (Better than a baby. Better than *my* baby, at any rate ...)

I had forgotten the pleasures of this kind of thing. What were my rituals? Those little daily reassurances that I gave to myself, as I might to a friend? Had I ever even had any? I had forgotten. It's easy to forget when you are constantly giving of yourself to another person – because even when they're not physically there, you are planning for them in your thoughts.

You are on high alert. You are poised to panic. Waiting for the alarm cry. It is an exhausting, self-nullifying state.

Jesca and I write in separate rooms and meet up for meal-times. We bathe leisurely, often three times a day, to refresh our heads. We smoke rollies, admiring the snow-capped mountains. We gather kindling in the woods and dry it out on top of the Rayburn stove. We dry our hair in front of the coal fire like fine Georgian ladies. We drink wine, sherry, whisky and chai tea she makes to her own recipe. I realise I have always liked routine. This is my kind of routine. I lie in bed until 9am reading every day, after waking of my own accord, which feels like the biggest luxury I have known for a long time – better than drinking champagne or travelling business on a plane.

I think about my son approximately every two and a half minutes. The guilt comes and goes. The worry comes and goes. I call home every day. I feel nourished and nurtured. That nourishment leads to much productivity. In four days I redraft a film script, write two TV pilots, a plan for this book, and ten pages of a new novel. By Saturday I am physically aching to see my son. But I also know I have done something I needed to do, for me. He is fine, with his dad and his grand-parents, and I will return refreshed and ready for another stint of hardcore mothering.

I thank Jesca and tell her how much good she's done me.

'Can't you buy the things you need with the baby, to remind yourself to self-care?' she says.

'No,' I reply instantly. And then I think about why. I say, slowly, 'The baby hates being in shops. He wants to get out. He cries. And when he cries, I still go into panic mode. Like the fight-or-flight part of my brain, the amygdala, starts pulsing, and I must leave immediately and give the baby exactly what he wants. I can't relax or focus on things I want.'

'Ohhhh,' Jesca says ominously. 'You have been reprogrammed.'

'Or, more accurately, I have been fucked up,' I reply.

But I also see that maybe I am blocking myself. Maybe I need to try.

Meanwhile, my writing routine has become one of daily adaptation, as I am living with someone who changes every day. That is a joyous thing and something we have to react to. I am so grateful to have my son in my life. But I cannot write when he is in the flat. Even when we are not in the same room, I know when he's awake. I know when he's upset. I know when he needs something. I am tuned in to his energy. I do not know how to break that frequency, and I am not sure I want to. My friend Nathan, an author, says: 'Your son doesn't give a shit about your book.' Which is absolutely true. And thank god for that. I don't have an office in the flat, but for the days he is at nursery, I have a desk in the corner of the lounge that faces the window, and along the windowsill I have precious trinkets that mark out the space as my space, and my space alone. When I look at them, and out of the window, I could be anyone anywhere, and that is the liberation a person needs to write. If a room of your own isn't possible, a view will do.

Postnatal depression aside, the remaining challenges of my writing life are not unique to motherhood. I am constantly trying to strike a balance between earning money, making things I truly love, spending time (and being present, not off in a fantasy) with the ones I love, keeping my mind and body healthy, having fun. I can't sod off for weeks on end in a motorhome around the Highlands, but I can go off for a week on my own here and there. I'm grateful for the things my son has brought to my writing, like the perspective to let some things go (especially at 5pm), and the skill to separate my work and home life more – which is never easy for a writer, or anyone self-employed. I am not saying you need a child to do this, and I want to be really careful about that, but this is what has happened in my specific circumstance, because of my child. It is strange and hard balancing two such utterly absorbing things: my child and my writing. I fail a lot, and things spill into each other, and there are arguments, and frustrations, and other such human occurrences. I am thankful for my husband's support, and for my son and my husband's gracious sharing of me with my work. Because they do share me with it. I love my work. I also know that without my work I am not myself. I can't be a good version of me, or a good mother, without it, because that communion between words on the page and my thoughts makes me feel well.

As I try to balance the various elements of my life every day, I appreciate that life is tidal. It moves forwards and backwards, forwards and backwards. It moves in and out. Depression, too, comes and goes like the tides. It's not something that passes through you and then is gone for ever. The tide comes from the middle of the Atlantic. A slack tide is where it stops, when it's about to turn.

Before I had a child I was a country; I was a culture. I had a language; spoken to me by me. I had secrets and a history and this land was a place to exist that I had carefully and lovingly built for myself. In this way it was totally, infinitely unique. And then something came and razed it to the ground. Decimated it. Suddenly, I had nowhere to be. I *was* nowhere. I was not only lost, I had lost myself. I was no longer able to be me with me. I think that is what can destroy a person. What I know now is there are ways to get this back – once you have accepted what has happened. Once you have shouted its name into the wind.

What I also know is that it was grief I was feeling, for everything I had and was before I became a mother. Grief for the life I had. Grief for my wildness. Grief for my queendom. The Kübler-Ross model denotes the five stages of grief as denial, anger, bargaining, depression and acceptance. I felt all of those. Grief is a funny thing to admit to when no one has died; when someone has, in fact, been born. But grief is about loss, not death. And I know now that there is a loss in any big life-change, even the ones you're grateful for. There is a grief that accompanies this loss. It is a grief that can coexist with the joy in your heart.

The Sun

I am healing and getting happier, and it feels like the world is slowly waking up to what women might need as they deal with the challenges of motherhood. An article published in the *Guardian* in 2019 featured a singing class designed for mums rather than babies. 'Melodies for Mums' is run by a not-for-profit social enterprise, Breathe, that aims to help new mothers with PND, or those at risk of it, and combat their symptoms by singing songs specially chosen to improve confidence and help them bond with their babies – songs like folk songs and gospel, sung in languages ranging from Hebrew to Zulu, often with three-part harmonies. Empowering stuff. A release of tension, too, perhaps. The focus on the mother is nice, even with the baby present in the group. In fact, making the mother's health story count is, I think, key to improving the postnatal experience for everyone, babies included.

The eminent British paediatrician and psychoanalyst Donald Winnicott said: 'There is no such thing as a baby' and 'a baby alone doesn't exist'. He meant that the baby cannot exist on its own, physically or psychologically. The baby and the person looking after it make a couple. It blows my mind that pregnant women have foetal DNA in their blood, and after you have a baby, their cells stay inside you for years. This connection is profound and physical.

Research in 2019 by the not-for-profit social enterprise Breathe Arts Health Research has already found that mothers with moderate to severe symptoms of PND who did group singing saw a faster improvement in their symptoms than a control group. A study of Melodies for Mums will test the impact and mechanisms involved further, with academics measuring women's levels of the stress hormone cortisol and the 'love hormone' oxytocin to assess bonding with their babies, and evaluate levels of depression, anxiety, coping, loneliness and social support. Since the programme began two years ago in Southwark, south-east London, 150 women have taken part. Now it is being expanded to reach hundreds more, as the sessions become part of a big study into how arts interventions boost physical and mental health, and how they could be scaled up to become NHS treatments.

'There's a wealth of anthropological and psychological research on the benefits of singing for individual mental health, mother–infant interactions and infant development,' says Daisy Fancourt, associate professor of psychobiology and epidemiology at UCL, and one of the leaders of the Melodies for Mums research. A recent study with older people in Kent found group singing had a significant effect on mental health and quality of life, including reducing anxiety, depression and loneliness.

I asked Rebecca Moore what women can do to heal after childbirth and ease themselves into new motherhood.

'As well as talking therapy [and] medication, there are tons of things we can do to heal,' she insists. 'Look at all areas of your life holistically. What you're eating can have a huge impact, which is difficult when you're a new mum because often you're just eating junk food and sugary stuff to feel awake. There are some supplements that can help. Exercise is helpful for depression, anxiety and trauma. Realistic exercise for a new mum could be to have a walk around the park for 15–20 minutes.

'Reconnecting with your body is important and not something we talk about. You might have new scars, or feel your body let you down or failed you. Also trauma can be held bodily so a lot of people will present, not saying they feel low, but with headaches or IBS or pain – and that can be a way that people tell us they are struggling. Things like scar massage can be really healing. Journaling trauma can help – if they can't yet say their story but can write it down. There is scientific evidence that journaling reduces trauma symptoms.

'Peer groups are really important – whether you find that in a phoneline, on Twitter, in a WhatsApp group … There are lots of great social media accounts putting out great information and breaking down a lot of taboos around motherhood. Trying to build social networks is important in terms of support. Loneliness can really impact on mental health. It's not easy to build those groups. Some people hate baby groups. The narrative is you'll suddenly have all these mummy friends and it will be great – in the park, with the sun shining – and it's not like that for most people. It'd be great if we could map that out for people antenatally: Who do you like to see? Who makes you feel great? Can you book in to see them once a month? What do you enjoy doing? What do you feel comfortable doing?

'What I want women to have is all the choices and then you pick the two or three from that list that work for you.'

For me, reconnecting with my body was key, through exercise. I now love running and do it whenever I can. I've never been into running before, but now I really appreciate the boost of endorphins it gives me. I won't be an exercise bore, but if you don't run and you feel down or stressed, try it. I find it really helps with writing, too – pushing myself forwards through space, with the world passing by on either side in my peripheral vision, that literal unspooling. I've untangled a lot of knotty plot points through running.

I also do yoga and I'm trying transcendental meditation. Well, if it's good enough for David Lynch …

My regular yoga teacher, Yagna, spent eight years living on an ashram in India, although she's originally from Germany and every now and then her six-year-old daughter comes into the room and reminds everyone that Yagna's original name is Evie. We practise at her flat in Hove, usually me and four or five other women. A few strange things happen to me there over the years; things that tell me my mind and body are getting back in touch. One time, I am moving my arm through the air in a movement and feel my hand pass through an area of thick, liquid warmth, as if through a ball of warm water suspended in the air. I gasp. Yagna asks what the matter is. I tell her. She smiles. 'That is energy,' she says.

Another session, Yagna asks us to think of a phrase, a few words, to use as a mantra as we do our practice. *Success and happiness*, I chant loudly in my mind, because those are the things I want the most. But as I'm moving from position to position, I find that my brain changes the words. They are not 'success and happiness' any more. They are 'patience and kindness'. I start to cry, pretending that the yoga has given me a blissful release – and in a way it has. Those words come louder because, even though they are not overtly what I want, they are the things I need more. My brain knows it.

Finally, Yagna asks us to do a visualisation exercise at the end of class. I go along with it, but I don't expect much. I'm not a big fan of visualisations – just seems like a waste of good sexual fantasy time. Yagna asks us to visualise a natural entity like a flower or a body of water or a heavenly body. I find myself picturing a tree. It is a beautiful tree – a blossom tree – thick with pink blooms, bowing over a lake to admire its reflection. *What a gorgeous cherry blossom I am*, the tree is thinking. I can't help but agree. Then, the water turns into a rushing river, and the tree can't see its reflection any more. The tree is chopped into hundreds of pieces that fall to the ground. A few pieces travel down the river, and one of them reaches a bank and takes root. It grows into another tree, a new tree, still beautiful with blossoms, but instead of looking over a lake it offers patches of shade that people come and have picnics in. A child comes and makes a swing on a low branch, and starts to swing back and forth.

When I tell Jesca about this vision, she says simply: 'The tree is you.'

I worry about how patriarchal this vision of mine is. Do I have to be useful and not narcissistic to be valued by society? Do women always have to be like that? Hmm. Or maybe it's just about giving yourself, sharing yourself, showing compassion and kindness ('patience and kindness'!) and getting more out of life that way.

What else have I learned? Don't separate friends into mum and non-mum camps. There is no mystery about shitty nappies. No more than any hangover. We have to smash the dichotomy of mums/non-mums, I think, to make progress.

I know that being maternal has nothing to do with actually physically being a mother. I've always been maternal – with my friends, sister, partners, cats, houseplants. Lately, with my parents. On good days, with myself. These are old skills I'm adapting, not new ones.

My son and I are very closely connected now. I long for him when we are apart. I want to kiss his feet every time I see them. I am obsessed with the biscuity smell of his scalp. I have pulled a muscle trying to make him laugh. A curl of his lip means he is going to lunge for the bath toy. He is mad for the water. They said he was too young for the underwater photo session I mistakenly took him to, but he went at the water four limbs thrashing, so they said he could try, and he aced it. 'He's broken the mould today, that one!' the photographer said.

It's a similar story at Baby Sensory. He lunges into the tunnel after the class leader says that babies are often afraid. Not mine. He is intrepid, impulsive and bold. He is my boy. I could explode with love for him. Every night I go into his room four or five times and check him as he sleeps, and every time I go in I whisper: 'We love you so much, you are safe, you never need to worry.' I want his dreams to be happy dreams.

When he is two, Ian and I decide to get tattoos – an act of solidarity and, for me, bodily ownership. We take a romantic day-trip to Canterbury to see a tattoo artist we love from Instagram. I already have tattoos but this is Ian's first.

I get a tattoo on my right forearm, on the inside part where it's smooth and flat and there are no freckles. It's a fox cub lying on a stack of books, with the words 'Be secret and exult' curled around it. It's a line of Yeats, from the poem 'To a Friend Whose Work Has Come to Nothing'. It feels apt, about making the work good for its own sake, and for my own sake. It is about being in my bubble, and loving being in my bubble, and seeing the value of my bubble for me and my brain, even if my work were, like Yeats' friend's, to 'come to nothing'. I wanted to get that inked into my skin so that I could see it every day and be reminded. Process first. Parenting is like that, too. Your heart is out walking around the world on two legs, and there's nothing you can do about that. Other than tell that heart how to be strong.

I send my friend Sally a photo of my new tattoo. Sally is from the north-east and every time she texts me I hear it out loud in her accent. We used to stay up all night and sing karaoke in her kitchen in south Manchester. Now we text each other awestruck nature-porn rants during *Springwatch* or *Autumnwatch* – which is keeping it wild, in some ways. She sends me craft ales in the post and makes me laugh more than anyone I know. When she sees my new tattoo she texts:

MATE, THERE'S AN 'H' IN EXHULT

This makes me laugh a lot.

I am grateful to lots of things for my return to happiness, but it is my friends who give me back my sense of humour.

Cape Wrath

In February 2020, before coronavirus shuts the world down, I travel alone to the Highlands of Scotland in a motorhome to work on this book. I spend a week there, thinking and writing. I have had two miscarriages in four months, but I know I want to do it again. I want another child. I feel strong from what I have been through and what I have learned. I am determined to do things differently next time, be more careful, more demanding, more honest, kinder to myself.

On my trip I drive right to the top of the country, to Durness, next to Cape Wrath, the most north-westerly point in Britain, where the wind is wild and the sea is wilder. I park my van at the clifftop campsite that is closed for winter. The owner has said I can park for free, advising me to stick to the less blustery side of the site: advice I merrily ignore. There are no toilet facilities or shop but I have everything I need in the van. I love travelling like this, fast and lonely, amidst the elements. The drive is almost my favourite part. We stitch ourselves back together in all kinds of ways. Muscles and ligaments. Stitch, stitch, stitch. White lines on a road. Stitch, stitch, stitch. Words on a page. Stitch, stitch, stitch.

It is sunny. The motorhome casts a long, wide shadow. I stare out to sea. Nothing until Orkney, then Shetland, then the Arctic. Here I am, at the opposite end of the country to Brighton. The south coast is over 700 miles away.

The wind is strong up here. The sea roars. As the afternoon turns into evening, I watch people walk their dogs on the sands below. There are white horses on the sea, where the foam turns high and hard, spraying back, fighting its own fate. There is a ferocity in the weather – a ferocity that suits me. The rage remains, in some ways. Maybe it has always been a part of me, deep down. Maybe it always will be. I feel as though I am reconnecting with the person I used to be, and the person I am. I find solace, and not for the first time, in the words of the poet Mary Oliver. Constant happiness is not mandatory. Allow all the feelings. This is how we move, learn and grow. Growth is not a distraction from life; it is the definition of it.

The Uses of Sorrow

(In my sleep I dreamed this poem)

Someone I loved once gave me a
box full of darkness.

It took me years to understand that
this, too, was a gift.

On the drive up here I noticed things I have never noticed before, even though I have made this trip eight or ten times in the past few decades. The surname 'Mackay' is everywhere. Even the campsite and shop are owned by Mackays. Mackay is a Scottish clan name on my mother's side. She was born a 'Mackie', anglicised down the line. Just after the roads become single-track, the A-road skirts a mountain and a huge boulder with a brass sign nailed to it: 'Mackay County'. Maybe that's why I've always felt so at home here. It's literally in my DNA. The rusty gorse and bright blue lochs. That's my facial colour palette, right there. I decide I would like to die in the Highlands – a cigarillo in my hand as the ice wind blows through my thinning hair. Scatter my ashes out to sea, or send them out there in an Orkney beer bottle.

Ian sends me some photos of the buoy, the red one near the old pier. He has just got a paddleboard and has paddled out to see it. I suppose we both wanted to conquer it. Own it. This symbol of the night; the deep. When I saw the photos he'd sent me I felt victorious for both of us. That mystery was revealed – with all its scrapes, rust, algae and other flaws. A dirty great buoy. That's all it was.

On the clifftop at Durness, with the elements all around, I feel in my spiritual home, as though my spirit is back. The moon and the mountains are here. I am looking back and down and all around. I feel as I always feel here: old and new and big and small and lost and found. Inside my head, I feel like me again. I hope this book helps if you don't feel like you. You are not alone. There are people and organisations waiting to listen. Let's smash – *really smash* – the notion that we need to be perfect to be good enough. This is not an ending where women have to be sorted out. This is an ending where women can still be messy most days. This is a matriarchal narrative, if you will. One of flesh and blood and bones and bits, one that is growing and changing and pushing and fighting and moving. One that has arms as big as the sky and a heart as deep as the sea and a mouth as hot as hell. If you can add your voice, add it. If you can't, cling to us. We can carry you. We can carry all of us.

There is another feeling: a new one. As I sit at my little desk in the van's back lounge, looking out, I realise I have felt this feeling before, in planes. That moment after the initial ascent, through the weather, when the plane reaches its cruising height and there is that moment of golden serenity. It is almost as though the engines stop. It is like being outside of time and space, suspended there; motionless. Amongst the copper-tinged clouds, the whole world curving away, there is a wiry, visceral sense of eternity.

Back home in Brighton, coronavirus hits. During the first lockdown, we discover we are pregnant again, for the third time in six months. I don't want to get my hopes up. Meanwhile, the world around us disintegrates. The death toll goes up daily. There is grief everywhere – I identify it quickly as grief, grief in disguise; it comes for me in similar ways, I see and hear it in my friends. We are grieving the collective loss of the world as we knew it: hanging out, going out, enjoying daily normalities. These are like the losses in new motherhood – solitude, sleep, thinking time – but on a global scale. Everyone is scared. I am scared. I am convinced I will miscarry again. But the pregnancy sticks. As I make the final edits on this book it is November 2020 and I am due to have my second baby later this month. I can't tell you I'm not terrified about getting PND again. I can tell you I feel a lot more prepared than last time, and I am doing lots of things differently. I have found out so many things I want to share. Things that feel strengthening and enlightening. And I am willing to go around again, through the maelstrom of motherhood, which is something I never thought I'd say four years ago.

As for that storm – I have metabolised it. I have brewed it in my pot, and the steam rises up and up, past the mountain tops. Surviving an illness is a transformation. It is also a love story, played out by you and your body. Almost daily I find myself and my burgeoning frame, my precious cargo, pulled towards the sea. I waddle down on my watery ankles, hugging my coat around my stomach, beyond where it still buttons. I stand and breathe on the pebbled inclines of the Brighton shoreline, feeling the winter air sweeping in. I wait for my daughter. I wait for the sun, which I feel now to the bones of me. The light that always comes after the dark.

Thanks

To Mum, Dad, Grandma, Lucie, Dave, Charlie, Matilda.

To Pat and Colin Williams.

To everyone at Profile Books and Wellcome, especially Ellen Johl, Fran Barrie, Helen Conford and Graeme Hall for believing in this book and making it a real thing.

To my agent Clare Conville and all at C&W.

To Katie Battcock, Camilla Young and Nick Fenwick at Curtis Brown.

To Chris Smith at CAA.

To Alex Glew for the sausages, kale, love and general joie de vivre. Merci, chérie.

To Stef Lake, for helping me identify what might be wrong, and your own courage to call it.

To Katie Leatham, for enlightening therapy, and words that helped me heal.

To Rosemary Kennedy, for living above us and coming down to save us.

To my dear, clever, humour-saving friends: Sally Cook, Katie Popperwell, Alison Taylor, Maria Roberts, Nicola Mostyn, Sarah Tierney, Holly Smale, Jesca Hoop, Natalie O'Hara, Alexandra Heminsley, Jess Ruston, M. K. Trevaskis, Emily Powell, Sarah Brocklehurst, Romana Majid, Eden Keane.

To Anna Burtt, for so much brain-freeing babysitting. I love you, Suzy.

To Valerie Leevers for the gifts on the doorstep and the wise articles.

I am indebted to all the wonderful women I interviewed who are doing pioneering work investigating maternal mental health and who shared with me their thoughts and findings. These include Professor Hilary Marland, Dr Sarah Crook, Dr Jodi Pawluski and Dr Rebecca Moore. (Thank you also, Rebecca, for the 'Pregnant Princess; Postnatal Pauper' line.)

Thank you to Sara Campin of the Nourish App.

Thank you to the Arts Council of England for the grant which helped hugely in the finishing of this book during the pandemic.

To all the wonderful midwives in Brighton and Hove who supported and cared for me, and all the NHS staff in the hospitals and clinics – the sonographers, nurses, health-care assistants, health visitors, doctors, receptionists – thank you so much. I have more good memories than bad.

To Didi Craze especially, who made my daughter's birth and first months so much less stressful – your kind eyes and magical words helped me believe I could do it again very differently.

To all the women and men who got in touch after I shared my story in the *Guardian* in 2018 – thank you for your stories and your generosity. You made me think this book could be a good idea. If you're struggling right now, hang in there. There are some organisations listed in the next few pages. Talk to everyone you feel you can. You are not letting your baby down. You are not letting anyone down. The more we all talk about this the more we all learn about this, and it becomes less a thing to feel ashamed of and more a thing that we can demand more support for.

Finally, to my boys, Ian and LF. Ian – thank you for being my shipmate in the wildest seas, a true friend and my full-heart love. Now and for ever: no half measures. LF – thank you for being my greatest teacher already, for holding my hand as we grow, for reminding me who I am. As you said the other day: *It's 100,000 years since I was a baby*. And it is.

Resources, Social Media and Websites

Candice Brathwaite, *I Am Not Your Baby Mother: What it's like to be a black British mother* (Quercus, 2020)

Chelsea Conoboy, 'Motherhood brings the most dramatic brain changes of a woman's life', *Boston Globe*, 17 July 2018

Dr Sarah Crook, 'The Uses of Maternal Distress in British Society, c. 1948–1979'

Sinead Gleeson, *Constellations* (Picador, 2019)

Jenni Gritters, 'This is Your Brain on Motherhood', *The New York Times*, 5 May 2020

Professor Hilary Marland, 'Under the shadow of maternity: birth, death and puerperal insanity in Victorian Britain', *History of Psychiatry*, Vol. 23, no. 1, March 2012

Maggie Nelson, *The Argonauts* (Melville House UK, 2016)

Emily Oster, *Expecting Better* (Penguin Press, 2013)

WHO, *International Classification of Diseases*, 11th Revision (2018)

The following are fantastic resources for preparing yourself for pregnancy, labour and motherhood

The Positive Birth Book Visual Birth Plan Cards by Milli Hill allow you to build a flow diagram, and plan for a wide range of eventualities during labour and immediately after. Hill's book *The Positive Birth Book* (Pinter & Martin, 2017) is wonderful and reassuring, too.

Dr Jodi Pawluski makes a podcast called 'Mommy Brain Revisited' (@mommybrain.revisited) where she interviews scientists about their latest work in the field.

@natgeorgas, for parenting neurodiverse kids
@mothers.wellness.toolkit
@drmdc_paediatric_psychologist
@psychotherapy_mum
@womensmentalhealthdoc
@dark_side_of_the_mum
@_drboyd
@parenthoodinmind

For BAME Women
@abueladoula
@brownpsychologist
@fivexmore_
@_prosperitys
@ravideepkaur_
@blackfemaletherapists
@blackmamasmatter
@therapyforlatinx
@queerdoulas

Apps I love
www.thenourishapp.com
www.calm.com

The following support groups and charities can help with birth trauma and postnatal mental health

Make Birth Better (makebirthbetter.org) is a unique
    collective of parents and professionals dedicated to
    reducing the life-changing impact of birth trauma.

PANDAS (pandasfoundation.org.uk) is a UK charity
    offering peer-to-peer support for families suffering
    from pre- and postnatal mental illnesses. Use their
    website to find a support group near you.

Dads Matter UK (dadsmatteruk.org) is a free service that
    provides support for dads worried about or suffering
    from depression, anxiety or post-traumatic stress
    disorder (PTSD).

The Maternal Mental Health Alliance (MMHA,
    maternalmentalhealthalliance.org) is a coalition of
    UK organisations committed to improving the mental
    health and wellbeing of women and their children in
    pregnancy and the first postnatal year.

You can also go to the NHS website (nhs.uk) and enter
    your location for nearby support groups.

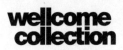

WELLCOME COLLECTION books explore health and human experience. From birth and beginnings to illness and loss, our books grapple with life's big questions through compelling writing and beautiful design. In partnership with leading independent publisher Profile Books, we champion essential voices and fresh perspectives across history, memoir, psychology, medicine and science.

WELLCOME COLLECTION is a free museum that aims to challenge how we all think and feel about health by connecting science, medicine, life and art. It is part of Wellcome, a global charitable foundation that supports science to solve urgent health challenges, working in more than seventy countries, with a focus on mental health, global heating and infectious diseases.

wellcomecollection.org